AMMA
The Ancient Art of Oriental Healing

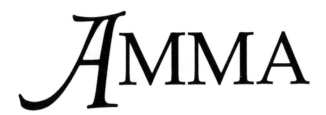

AMMA

The Ancient Art of Oriental Healing

by Tina Sohn as told to Donna Finando

with supplementary text by Robert Sohn and Steven Finando

Illustrations by Richard Rockwell

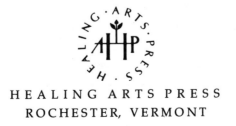

HEALING ARTS PRESS

ROCHESTER, VERMONT

Healing Arts Press
One Park Street
Rochester, Vermont 05767

LIBRARY OF CONGRESS CATALOGING IN PUBLICATION DATA

Sohn, Tina.
    Amma, the ancient art of Oriental healing/by Tina Sohn and Donna
Finando; illustrations by Richard Rockwell.
      p. cm.
    Includes index.
    ISBN 0-89281-233-8 (cloth).   ISBN 0-89281-229-X (pbk.)
    1. Massage. 2. Medicine, Chinese. 3. Holistic medicine.
I. Finando, Donna. II. Title.

RM723.C5S64   1988   88-5081
615.8′8′095—dc 19   CIP

Printed and bound in the United States

10 9 8 7 6 5 4 3 2 1

Healing Arts Press is a division of Inner Traditions International, Ltd.

Distributed to the book trade in the United States by Harper and Row Publishers, Inc.
Distributed to the book trade in Canada by Book Center, Inc., Montreal, Quebec
Distributed to the health food trade in Canada by Alive Books, Toronto and Vancouver

CONTENTS

How to Use This Book   *xi*

PART I. The Philosophy   *1*

   1. What Is AMMA Therapy?   *3*

   2. Wholistic Health   *7*

   3. The Homeodynamic Model of Health   *17*

   4. The Development of a Therapist   *26*

PART II. The Principles   *37*

   5. Introduction to Basic Oriental Anatomy and

      Physiology   *39*

PART III. The Practice   *111*

   6. The Hand   *113*

      An Anatomical Description

      Care of the Hands

   7. Hand Exercises   *123*

   8. Hand Techniques   *127*

   9. Principles of Treatment   *134*

  10. The Basic AMMA   *136*

FOREWORD

by Robert S. Mendelsohn, M.D.

MY first meeting with Tina Sohn convinced me that she knows something that American doctors do not, particularly since her healing technique relieved the pain and disability my wife had been suffering from a finger injury. Since then, I have had the opportunity to observe closely Mrs. Sohn's remarkable work.

Together with her husband, Dr. Robert Sohn, Mrs. Sohn founded and directs the Wholistic Health Center in Manhasset, New York. They have translated the principle that health means "to make whole" into the practical application of a variety of conventional and alternative healing strategies: nutritional analysis and instruction, stress reduction techniques, training in biofeedback, chiropractic, psychological counseling, acupuncture, and a highly specialized and significant therapeutic massage therapy called Amma.

It is Amma therapy that makes Mrs. Sohn unique. Amma is an ancient system of therapeutic massage that promotes health and well-being by circulating the body energies through muscular manipulation, draining the lymphatic system, and increasing the circulation within the cardiovascular system.

Mrs. Sohn's family has a long history of mastery in the healing and martial arts. Now, Tina Sohn has revitalized Amma therapy at the Wholistic Health Center. She has integrated her extensive training and her highly evolved, natural healing sensitivity into Amma, and has since trained all the senior Amma therapists at the Center.

As the American people's disappointment with modern medicine deepens, many are seeking therapies previously overlooked. Take my word for it—the Manhasset Wholistic Health Center is the best-kept secret in America today. This fine book reveals, for the first time, in a style easily understandable to the Western world, methods of achieving and maintaining health, validated not merely by evanescent modern science but by centuries of theoretical development and pragmatic application. Every professional in the health field must know about Amma therapy. But this book is not exclusively for professionals; this book is for everyone!

A COMMENT

by Bertram Spector, Ph.D.

AS one educated in allopathic medicine, I was some-what skeptical of the potential benefits of Amma therapy when first introduced to it at the Wholistic Health Center in Manhasset, New York. Some time earlier, following extensive tests at the Long Island Jewish Hospital which revealed severe curtailment of respiratory efficiency (coupled with hypertension), I sought conventional medical treatment. Unfortunately, little improvement was noticed after ten months. At that time Dr. Steven Finando introduced me to the wife of Dr. Robert Sohn, Tina Sohn, a leading expert in Eastern health therapies, especially Amma therapy.

After my first experience with Amma therapy, there was impressive improvement, and within a few weeks my respiratory capacities were back to normal. Concurrently, my hypertension, partially controlled by medication, was reduced to excellent normal levels.

Subsequently, a pituitary adenoma in the sella turcica, diagnosed by CAT scan at a leading medical center, regressed almost completely, as disclosed three months later in coned-down X rays, under the influence of combined Amma therapy by Tina Sohn, and acupuncture by Dr. Finando and Dr. Sohn.

Today, I am a firm believer in the powerful benefits of Amma therapy and acupuncture, when performed by experts, for many, otherwise insoluble, health problems, and for the maintenance of optimal well-being.

HOW TO USE
THIS BOOK

AMMA therapy is a highly advanced, extremely specific form of manipulative therapy. As with all great forms of health care, a fundamental *idea* of the manner of application can be ascertained from a book. However, the serious student must have a teacher, a competent guide, to provide direction in the subtleties of the art. Teaching can take place in a private setting, or as part of a formal program of study; but you must have a teacher to guide you in your endeavors to become skillful in this great art. This is a text book. It was designed for the serious student of Amma who needs a guide for reference or a study guide for practice, while learning the fundamental principles and techniques. Practice, of course, is most beneficial with a partner. Study must be accomplished by yourself.

Maximum benefit will be attained if you adhere to the following guidelines while studying this book:

1. Study, and seek to understand through consistent thought, the nature of the energy system and the physiology of each organ channel as presented.

2. Learn the pathways of the Channels as they flow throughout the body. You should be able to readily locate and trace the surface pathways, the Tendino-Muscle Pathways, and the cutaneous regions on the body. This knowledge is employed in all phases of the practice of Amma therapy.

3. Develop the essential hand and arm strength by practicing the specially developed hand exercises in Chapter 8. Practice the exercises daily. Do not feel satisfied with any gain in strength and flexibility, as there is always more to be attained. Only after developing a high degree of physical strength can more subtle sensitivities begin to appear.

4. Continually practice relaxation techniques, for in such activities lies the path toward true accomplishment as a healing sensitive. When there is true relaxation of the fingers, hands, arms, shoulders, chest, belly, back, perineum, legs, and feet, your treatments will produce vitality in both your patients and yourself that is unparalleled in other healing modalities. With relaxation comes the free flow of *qi* that is ultimately used by the advanced practitioner of Amma therapy to promote the healing of patients.

5. Practice the hand techniques conscientiously until they are as natural and instinctive as the use of the hands in eating, washing, and turning pages. These techniques are employed in the Basic Amma as well as in the more advanced forms of Amma therapy.

6. Familiarize yourself completely with the Basic Amma as it is presented. Learn it and practice it until it can be performed with ease and fluidity of motion. This will take many months of practice.

7. Above all, practice. It will be months before comfort is attained in executing the Basic Amma, and years before true accomplishment in this takes place. This is not a simple bodywork technique—it is an art of great power. Sensitivity to another's body and energy is a subtle and wonderful gift. Work at it and it will be yours.

PART ONE

The Philosophy

CHAPTER ONE
What is Amma Therapy?

AMMA therapy is an ancient healing system whose origins date back approximately 5,000 years to the period of the Yellow Emperor. Amma is a complex and highly refined system of bodywork therapy employing a wide variety of massage techniques, manipulations, and the application of pressure, friction, and touch to points and the channels on which they are found. The channels are the pathways through which energy passes throughout the body.

Many theories have been suggested regarding the origins of Amma therapy that generally take an evolutionary position. That is, in early civilizations primitive people naturally sought to relieve pains by rubbing the body. The evolutionary position holds that Amma evolved from early experimentation with rubbing. Hence the name. Am-ma means "push-pull" in Chinese. However, the extreme sophistication of Amma makes such theories doubtful. The "evolutionary" position is one that *assumes* evolution, while in the case of Amma and many other traditions of the Orient, devolution seems much more likely. The Amma that has been practiced in modern China or Japan seems to be a devolved version of the art, in which the basic massage techniques are used exclusively. The subtlety and power of Amma was lost. Perhaps our ancestors were more in touch and aware of their bodies and could feel the flow of energy in their systems. Such a possibility could explain the precise delineation of acupuncture points and the knowledge of the specific effects of such points on the physiology. It is important to note that Oriental physicians generally never saw the inside of the human body. The ancient texts of the "inner" or "soft" styles of the martial arts all seem to indicate an awareness, sensitivity, and subtlety that is rarely found in practitioners of these arts today. Our egos may reject the idea that earlier societies were in some ways more advanced than our own, but such an explanation seems coherent with what we know about all the Oriental arts concerned with the subtle energies of living systems.

All arts, especially those that involve great attention to detail, extraordinary sensitivities, kinesthetic awareness, and control, are quite difficult to teach to others. The result is often a disintegration of the art, whereby the lower or more superficial forms of the original practices are taken on by the student. The intent of this book is to serve as the first of several texts and references for the serious student and practitioner, to revitalize the practice of the ancient forms of Amma, and to offer to the student the means of attaining the more subtle skills and sensitivities. It is, of course, the responsibility of the student himself to practice what is given. As sensitivity and awareness grow, so will the effectiveness and beauty of the practice of Amma therapy, and Amma will regain the respect it had in the ancient years as the primary modality of healing.

It is interesting to note that Amma therapy utilizes all the techniques of the major forms of therapeutic massage. Deep pressure and point manipulation used in Shiatsu massage are applied in the administration of an Amma treatment by the master practitioner to attain the desired effects of energetic movement and release of muscular contraction. Foot reflex points, commonly referred to as "foot reflexology," are stimulated during the course of a treatment. Stimulation of these points often has profound results on the deeper organs and tissues of the body. Deep fascial manipulation techniques and connective tissue manipulation used in Rolfing are part of the repertoire of the master therapist, as well as the muscle stretching and pushing techniques that are commonly used in the European or Swedish massage. In addition, the master therapist is well versed in, and fully capable of, the skeletal manipulations that are the basis of chiropractic. Amma therefore is less defined by a specific technique than by its purpose, philosophy, and sophisticated practice as a healing art.

It is probable that Amma was actually the grandparent of traditional Chinese medicine. It is fundamentally an energetic therapy concerned with the balance and movement of "life energy" in the human body.[1] From the basic application of hand techniques used to balance the flow of energy, other methods were developed, including the use of needles (acupuncture), heat (moxibustion), skeletal manipulations, the appropriate use of herbal medications, diet, and meditation. In traditional Chinese medicine all these approaches are concerned with the flow and balance of energy in the channels. The modern Amma therapist is knowledegable in all of these areas, but relies primarily on the sensitivity and strength of the hands to manipulate life energy.

The training of an Amma therapist emphasizes the personal development of the individual. Physically, great strength must be developed so that precise pressures can be applied without strain. Muscular endurance must also evolve so that patients may be treated without fatigue. Physical strength must be accompanied by muscular control and kinesthetic awareness to provide the subtle differences in manipulative techniques that are necessary within the context of the treatment. All movements must be executed from the proper portions of the hand without unnecessary strain on other muscle groups. Consider the fact that in acupuncture a great deal of attention is given to the type of needle used, its angle and depth of insertion, and a wide variety of manipulations of the needles necessary to effect maximum benefits. To achieve the proper effects of point application by the hand requires an awareness of pressure, angle, force vectors, and several other variables.

Sensitivity plays a fundamental role in Amma. First, the practitioner must combine anatomical knowledge with the ability to palpate so that origins and insertions of muscles can be located, as well as bone protuberances, sutures, and other anatomical "landmarks" necessary for practice. However, this sensitivity must extend to the more evolved ability to locate with precision the superficial pathways of the channel system and points on these pathways. This requires a level of awareness and sensitivity that is tuned to the energy system. Amma therapy actually goes beyond the use of the fourteen major channels, or energy pathways, and makes use of the lesser known Tendino-Muscle and Connecting Channels as well. The Amma therapist must be prepared to feel extremely subtle changes in the skin as well as in the deep muscle layers. It is important to note that all the Amma therapists at the Wholistic Health Center practice Hatha Yoga and T'ai Chi Chuan to develop sensitivity and the ability to control the energy that flows within their own bodies. Ultimately, the therapist develops the ability to use this *qi* to help heal others. Amma can be a means of enormous personal development for the practitioner.

The ability to heal another is fundamentally unattainable without great self-awareness and inner self-control. A basic aspect of the development of a true Amma therapist must be the development of control of his own inner emotional nature. When one is bound to his emotional experience and to the pictures and ideas that one has of himself, as opposed to the reality of oneself, one can not help another. Guidance is needed to break through the veils of fantasy. In the attempt to become an Amma therapist, a competent guide must be sought out and his guidance followed in all areas of direction, physical as well as emotional.

The exercises in this book are used by Mrs. Sohn and in the training of Amma therapists of the New Center for Wholistic Health Education and Research. They represent exercises that the students found most beneficial and helped to prepare them for the rigors of using Amma therapy. The basic treatment offered here is the groundwork for all the treatments that have been used on thousands of patients at the Wholistic Health Center in Manhasset, New York, and was taught as Mrs. Sohn defined it. In part, this book is an attempt to codify and preserve an ancient healing art as taught by one of its few masters in the world. It is hoped that this text will be a valuable guide for the professional and the student of manipulative therapies.

Endnote   [1] The idea of "life energy" or vital force is an ancient concept of Eastern healing arts. It is called *qi* in China, *ki* in Japan, and *pran* in India. It was first investigated in the West through Kirlian and infrared photography and electrical conductance.

CHAPTER TWO

Wholistic Health

AT the turn of the century, as civilized society began to move through the exciting and often painful birth process of the technological era, the development of objective methods of investigation was dominating scientific thought. This was not a sudden event, but a logical result of many forces. The early work of Galileo and Descartes, and the work of physical scientists through the time of Newton, represented the movement toward an intelligent attempt to systematically uncover mathematical relationships governing physical processes. Medicine and biology demonstrated a long historical movement toward a more objective, systematic exploration of nature. Harvey, Darwin, Pasteur, and many others led the way toward the seeking of truth unencumbered by the dogma of religion. The refreshing winds of new discovery, unleashed by scientific method, carried the sciences toward seeking more objective methods in the search for knowledge. It is important to note that concomitant with the development of the sciences there was a fragmentation of the Western church, and a weakening hold by organized religion. After centuries of explanations provided by religious leaders based upon "God's Will," a rebellion, swelling over two centuries, began to take place. It is characterized as a negation of the spiritual and a deepening involvement with the material. A major force for the development of the materialist viewpoint was the advent of the industrial and technological revolution. As never before, technology provided the means for exploration of the material world. As the technology became available, physicists studied the nature of matter by attempting to break it down into its component parts, studying the properties of molecules, atoms, and subatomic particles. Physicists were studying inanimate matter (later discovered to be extremely animate) by reducing it to its most fundamental pieces. As technology evolved and physicists entered previously unexplored territories, great discoveries of atomic structure sped the advancement of technology. Yet, we are still far from understanding the fundamental nature of matter.

Physics has always led the other sciences. As systematic methods of study were evolved by physicists, other sciences sought to establish greater rigor in experimentation. The biological sciences, with the rapid development of exploratory technologies, began to adapt scientific method to the study of life. However, the method mimicked physics, and sought to use advancing technology to study life by breaking it down into smaller and smaller structural units. This approach gave primacy to biological structure, and ultimately viewed function as a consequence of structure. As a result, there has been enormous technological development associated with this approach, and a greater understanding of biological mechanisms, but hardly a greater comprehension of the nature of life. Something was lost by looking at life microscopically: by losing the awareness of the relationship between microcosmos and macrocosmos, thereby losing sight of the miracle of a living organism. Like all great historical movements that were reactions to confined modes of thinking, the new surge toward materialism went to extremes. Scientific thought was directed to what could be measured, and the new technology provided new "rulers" and "scales" with great rapidity.

The biological and natural sciences were then followed by the field of psychology. It seems strange to consider psychology, the study of the psyche, as a materialist study. Psychology had classically been part of the departments of philosophy at the universities. It was considered a branch of philosophy. Instead of adapting the use of scientific method to the study of psychology, behaviorism became the dominant force of modern psychology, to the extent that psychology declared itself a science and sought to provide objective measurement to human behavior. Behaviorists reached extremes where they felt that only observable phenomena were worthy of study. The result was a concept of human psychology that was measured by IQ scores, latency of responses, and learning rates, but was grossly indifferent to the internal world of the human psyche. The behavioral approach was an attempt to study smaller and smaller units of behavior and establish, if possible, mathematical relationships to measure and predict behavior.

Certainly this provides an interesting tool for study, but it is extremely limited in its concept of the human being. We have not yet passed beyond materialist thinking in psychology. The ultimate extreme of materialist psychological investigation is the idea that there is no dichotomy between mind and body because the mind *is* the body! Brain researchers are functioning under a model that is the ultimate and expected end of the structural viewpoint: that the brain, neurons, neurological activity, and loci of the brain *are* the mind, and the mind has no existence separate from the structure of an organ. It was in this atmosphere of scientific accomplishment and technological advances that materialistic thinking was most seriously advanced. It provided the advantage of breaking with traditions and viewpoints that sought to silence discovery and new thought, but, like most powerful tools, it carried a second edge that looked at things in completely structural ways, and provided a new type of blindness to twentieth-century thought.

This attempt to apply the methodology of the physical sciences to the biological and psychological sciences is called *reductionism*. Reductionists assumed that by breaking things down into smaller and smaller pieces, greater understanding of the "thing" would result. While this approach obviously produced information, the concept of reductionism began to present clear problems when applied to biological, psychological, and medical sciences. It resulted in a structural, rather than functional, approach to understanding life, and the dynamic, interactive quality of life processes was relegated to a small place in medical practice. Organs are now removed, nerves severed, and powerful pharmaceuticals administered with little understanding of the consequences of such radical actions on the delicate biosystem of the living body. Further, by evolving sharp delineations between psychology and medicine, an artificial model of the human being was created.

Reductionism is attractive, since it clearly lends itself to what we call the "scientific" approach to knowledge and understanding. The twentieth century has been dominated by this approach, perhaps in reaction to centuries of superstition, quackery, and church-dictated "truth." Technological development provided the tools for building the foundation of the most rapidly changing society in recorded history. As is the case with any new direction, there tended to be a pendulum effect that swings to an extreme, often disregarding anything old, regardless of its value. With rapid technological development, the ancient wisdom of man's part in the ecosphere was ignored, and only in recent years have we been forced to face the tragic effects of this mistake. We are now facing a crisis in health, evidenced by the combination of the rapid decline of

infectious disease with the enormous rise in degenerative disease processes that allows longer life for more people—a longer
life that is often painful, crippling, and degrading. Is it possible that historians will look back upon the relatively short
history of reductionist-based medicine, and see a great mistake, a folly as dangerous as medieval bleeding?

Our health care delivery system reflects the reductionist bias
in its orientation toward technological and mechanistic
methods of caring for human beings. The extremes of these
approaches have led to the nightmare of an extraordinarily
complex, expensive, and specialized health care system;
mechanistic manipulations in surgery receive far greater
emphasis than how to eat and exercise properly. The miracles
of modern medicine are accompanied by a series of medical
abuses, ranging from insensitivity and dehumanizing behav-
iors to mortally destructive actions. Technological societies
have embraced reductionist thinking to such a point that modern medicine, less than two hundred years old (less than fifty
years old is more accurate, since medicine as we know it today
began with the development of antibiotics), is now considered
the medicine, losing sight of health care methodologies that
have endured, with good reason, for thousands of years.
Many people have forgotten that what is now called medicine
is really just one approach to health care: one that has value,
but one among many.

In response to reductionist thinking, a rather ancient concept was resurrected and given the name "(w)holism."[1] The
philosophy of wholism does not refute the potential value of
reductionist thinking, but simply reminds us that "the whole is
greater than the sum of its parts." This important idea for
health care affirms the need to understand human health from
a broad perspective. Human beings are not a collection of
organs, muscles, bones, and nerves, but represent something
far more complex, integrating many systems that result in an
ongoing dynamic being. Human beings have physical, emotional, intellectual, and metaphysical lives that are intertwined
and defy reductionist examination. In addition, human beings
are part of the cosmos. They do not exist in a vacuum. Each
person exists within a physical, psychological, and spiritual
environment that is crucial to understanding the meaning of
individual health. It is interesting to note that the word "heal"
means "to make whole." To understand health, one must have
some understanding of the whole. The willingness to understand health from this wide perspective, including reductionist information, is the basis of wholistic health care. Wholistic

health shares a great deal with Chinese Taoist philosophy. Tao may be translated as "the Way," referring to "the way of all things." The course of living that is in harmony with "the Way" is the way of health. That which opposes the Tao leads to *disease*.[2] Wholistic health care seeks to work in harmony with "the Way." It is obvious that comprehension of the Tao is not something attainable by understanding the minutae of cellular structure, but requires at least an ecological perspective of human health. This requires consideration of many intangibles connected to the quality of life and the delicate balances of the human condition that are affected by factors that include human relationships, aspirations, and a rapidly changing society. It is clear that the old boundaries between physical and psychological health must be radically altered.

One obvious principle of wholistic health is that mind and body really cannot be differentiated, but must be seen as a single entity, engaged in an ongoing dynamic called *life*. There cannot be a psychological problem that does not have a physiological effect, with the reverse holding equally true. Every student of basic physiology knows of the subtle physiological responsiveness of the human being. The GSR (galvanic skin response) measures subtle changes of electrical conductivity on the skin surface. Major reactions can be observed when a human being hears a word like "snake." This means that there is a constant dynamic between cognitive and physiological processes, a never-ending interaction between mind and body that obliterates any clear distinction between the two and questions whether there can even be a realistic conception of a dichotomy. A moment of reflection demonstrates this relationship. Heart attack, with all the associated problems of hypertension, coronary artery disease, and so on, is highly connected with stress and one's psychological life. There are countless studies about the Type A individual and the stress factors of modern life. Thus far, physicians have even come to suggest that their patients "take it easy," or go on vacation, but far too often they resort to their prescription pads for solutions. Such "solutions" have made drugs like Valium among the most widely used medications in the world. We are the most drugged and drug-abusive society in history, precisely because of a recognition of the negative effects of stress, but with a concomitant desire for a quick and easy solution. In addition, we are aware of how disease affects us psychologically, with associated feelings of anxiety, depression, lethargy, hyperactivity, or hyper-reactivity.

Wholism advances the concept of the *mindbody*, a concept

that is far more reflective of the human reality than an arbitrary division of mind and body. This means that there are diseases of the mindbody, treatments for the mindbody, and methods of maintaining the health of the mindbody. This concept not only expresses the unity of mind and body, but expresses the interactive nature of the human: the fact that it is impossible to treat a heart, or arm, or lung, isolated from the dynamic of a living being. It is precisely in the simple fact that we are concerned with the health of a person, a human being, rather than a body part that wholism begins to differentiate its approach to health care.

In providing treatment, the wholistic practitioner seeks to follow a Taoist principle that was eloquently expressed by Hippocrates: "First do no harm." By taking a broad view of health, the wholistic practitioner recognizes that many cures are worse than the disease. Indeed, with the advent of technology and more potent pharmaceuticals, iatrogenic (physician-caused) disease has become a major issue of modern health care. An examination of the ten top-selling prescription drugs includes a list of narcotics, diuretics, anti-inflammatories, and many others, that all have potentially dangerous side effects. In 1982, a study done at Harvard University attempted to ascertain whether physicians prescribed drugs based upon research papers or as a function of advertising by the pharmaceutical manufacturers. The study found that while physicians thought they were most influenced by research, their actual prescribing practices included drugs that were ineffective or had no value for the conditions for which they were prescribed. This information was available in well-documented research, yet the prescribing went on according to how the drugs were advertised. Iatrogenic problems are common because the view of a human being as a compartmentalized, structural phenomenon does not see the enormous potential damage of invasive methods on a carefully balanced biological system.

Wholistic health care tends to minimize iatrogenic problems because it approaches human beings, the mindbody, with an almost religious awe. The recognition of the exceedingly complex nature of living things, and the extraordinary web of interactive processes that are involved in health, precludes the casual use of pharmaceuticals and invasive therapies. It requires a broader perspective of human health and a larger conception of time than the simplistic "kill-the-symptom" view of health. Wholism sees the most profound power of health and healing to be inherent in the mindbody. Therefore, wholistic health practice seeks to support and encourage healing, rather than force it whenever possible. Such practice seeks natural, safe, minimally invasive methods to help the mindbody to heal itself. Practitioners of wholistic health tend to see themselves as agents or catalysts of the healing process, rather than as the source of healing. Much wholistic health practice is directed toward education and the removal of sources of abuse to our health. Unfortunately, this, too, can be taken to extremes; when a patient is in an extremely critical, life-threatening situation, it may be necessary to use invasive, perhaps even dangerous procedures. Modern medicine is encompassed by the practice of wholistic health, but its application is often limited to the treatment of problems that are in advanced stages, or most effectively treated by modern methods. Modern medical doctors often find a major role as diagnosticians in wholistic health, with a minor part to play in providing treatment, because of the "disease" rather than "health" orientation of the medical model.

Actually, the concept of treatment must be expanded when it is applied to wholistic health. The relationship between patient and practitioner is not the "just do as I say" (and often "not as I do") relationship that is so well known in health care. Both the patient and practitioner must "care" in wholistic health. Wholistic approaches to health emphasize changes in lifestyle, education, and overall patient responsibility. Patients must recognize that they are ultimately responsible for their own health and well-being based on a cooperative effort with a professional. In seeking health, an individual must understand that he or she has to take an active role in the process: learning, making changes in daily habits, and eating and exercising properly. The potential of wholistic health care is actualized only when an individual moves from being a passive recipient to becoming an active participant in health development. The wholistic practitioner has an additional responsibility beyond providing care and information. He must also serve as a model of the process. Obese, smoking, stressed, and sedentary health professionals are living a lie. In ancient China, acupuncturists did not treat a patient if the acupuncturist wasn't feeling well. A sickly physician was an impossibility. This role of a health professional is often minimized by people in the healing arts, but it is actually crucial in providing the patient with support and trust in the process. In addition, there is an enormous difference between being told about smoking, nutrition, and exercise by a practitioner who practices and understands what is expressed, and being told about a series of rules by a practitioner with no experience in their application.

The disease orientation of the medical model is demonstrated in its focus on the treatment of disease conditions rather than on the promotion of health. Preventative medicine is certainly part of the medical model, but the billions of dollars spent each year on medical costs are not for preventative measures. Insurance companies often reflect this bias, paying the costs for lung surgery but refusing payment for a program to help stop smoking. Fortunately, this is changing, but mostly because of obvious economic motivations. Most people see a doctor only when they are ill, rather than working with a professional to develop their health to its maximum potential. Wholistic health care is health-oriented. It seeks to avoid serious problems and prevent disease more than to alleviate symptoms quickly. It is easier to maintain health, making minor adjustments in behavior as necessary, than to apply drastic intervention once the system has deteriorated to a serious condition. This is why the major "treatment" in wholistic health is education. Methods of treatment such as acupuncture, Amma therapy, chiropractic, and biofeedback are necessary to help an individual return to health, but without concomitant changes in lifestyle, such therapies face an ongoing battle with illness.

Perhaps the single most distinguishing characteristic of wholistic health is that it conceives of human beings in a way that is radically different from that of modern medicine. Medicine, reflecting the reductionist viewpoint, sees the body in a materialistic way. Such a view sees human beings like machinery, where parts break down or systems cease to function, and the solution lies in the replacement of worn parts, lubrication, or overriding a system that isn't functioning. This is connected to the structural view, whereby only repair or interference with structure is the basis of health care. A radically different and wonderfully complementary concept of health care is the functional orientation that dominates the health care of the East. The wholistic model sees a human being as an energy system that controls and directs all physical functioning. Disruptions in the flow of this energy result in disease; physical or psychological stresses often cause disruption of this energy. The energy model unifies and explains the other principles of wholistic health care, explaining the need for a mindbody concept, or why minimal intervention is important in treating disease. The disastrous effects of many medications and "simple" surgical procedures on the energy system over time is only beginning to be seen in the increasing number of iatrogenic problems. Many procedures, such as the indiscriminate use of steroids, simply mask symptoms while intensifying the problem and weakening the immune system. Wholistic health sees the energy system as a priori to the physical system, and that must be understood to attain real health. The energy system, composed of antagonistic or opposing forces, must remain in a state of balance if health is to be maintained. Imbalance results in disease. The implications of the human being as an energy system are profound, and must be explored in terms of human relationships, the effects of practitioner and patient interactions, the quality of food and exercise, and, ultimately, the relationship between the individual and the cosmos. As material bodies, we are individual beings, separate and distinct from one another. As energy fields, we are highly interactive and connected.

Wholism was a reaction to the materialistic viewpoint of modern physics and its application of reductionism as the fundamental method of study. It is ironic that from such reduction of matter to finer and finer particles, and with increasing technological development, modern physics has entered the world of subatomic, or particle, physics. Now the leading researchers in nuclear physics are providing a very different message: there is no material universe. There is only energy, or movement: only vibration. In addition, such energy does not exist as an independent phenomenon but as a result of highly complex interactions between forces. Physics is coming to the viewpoint that the universe is a highly interactive matrix of energies, each influencing the other in both direct and subtle ways. Bell's theorem suggests that the universe is completely interconnected, with events influencing each other without any restrictions on distance. Einstein demonstrated the primacy of energy and the nonmaterial nature of reality. Other theorists offer similar notions of matter coming in and out of existence in a multidimensional matrix of reality. Since physics has historically spearheaded the directions of study taken by the the other sciences, it is possible that the reductionist-materialist-structuralist viewpoint is already outdated. The new psychology, physiology, and medicine will be wholistic-energetic-functional. Of course, as we move in such a direction, we will only come to rediscover the truths that have existed for millenia, and it is hoped, return to a place of greater rationality, humanism, and consciousness.

Endnotes

[1] Briefly stated, *holism* is a philosophical principle that expresses the idea that the whole is greater than the sum of its parts. In recent years the spelling has been modified by individuals and organizations that are committed to the principles of health care and health maintenance, to emphasize the idea of "whole." The spelling *wholism* has become popular and is now an alternative spelling of the word.

[2] Disease is defined in the *American Heritage Dictionary* as "an abnormal condition of an organism or part, especially as a consequence of infection, inherent weakness or environmental stress that impairs normal physiological function." In common parlance, disease is considered a pathologic disturbance, or illness. The meaning of disease is expanded here to include its literal meaning: "dis-ease: the lack, or absence, of ease." With respect to health care, dis-ease is an extremely common experience. What people experience as "normal physical function" is very often dis-ease: ongoing constipation, recurrent headache, chronic backache. We make the distinction between disease and dis-ease to emphasize the lack of real health in the general population today and the need for the practices that will lead to well-being in health.

CHAPTER THREE
The Homeodynamic Model

THE bodily condition in which there is a balanced and harmonious functioning of all physiological activity is called homeostasis, or "steady state." The complex biochemical, neurological, and mechanical processes that constitute human physiology are all directed toward the maintenance of a delicate equilibrium that characterizes health. However, to emphasize the extremely dynamic nature of this process, and to differentiate it from the more encompassing idea of energetic balance, the term "homeodynamic" will be used. "Homeodynamic" emphasizes the ongoing balance resulting from activating and depressing functions that exists between the various organ systems. It is this active process of constant correction that most reflects the energy system in a state of health, and as such, the term "homeodynamic" may better define this balance. A good analogy to the homeodynamic mechanism is the tightrope walker, who is constantly making subtle corrections as any loss of balance begins to occur.

Energy moves through the body along complex pathways or channels according to certain daily and seasonal "tides." This energy serves to regulate the functions of the various organs and physiological processes. Acupuncture is based upon the treatment of specific points along these channels. Amma is directed toward the treatment of the channels as well as the points located on them. When energy of the proper quality is moving through the system in a balanced, harmonious way, a person is considered to be in a state of health, reflected as a state of vitality, stability, and well-being. When the system ceases to be in a state of balance, *dis-ease* begins to be manifest, first being reflected in minor ailments and then in more serious symptoms. The homeodynamic model of health seeks to establish a balanced flow of energy and to remove all sources of imbalance. The concept requires understanding the various sources of imbalance as well as the various means for restoring harmony. It is important to remember that the system will naturally tend toward homeodynamic balance and maintain that balance unless a source of interference is present. In this way, the mindbody can be seen as a microcosm of an ecosphere, with complex relationships providing a check and balance system to maintain internal harmony. As we have frequently seen, ecological balance can be drastically affected by what appear to be minor disturbances of the system. The far-ranging consequences of what may appear to be unrelated events can often be disastrous. Because the homeodynamic model is functionally, rather than structurally, based, it is extremely interactive: the effect on one component of the model has extensive effects in other areas. For example, an apparent structural problem inducing a mild sciatica can also interfere with energy associated with the genitourinary system, and result in problems months later. It is therefore important that energetic imbalances be corrected, and when possible, the sources of such imbalances must be corrected as well.

There are many possible sources of imbalance in the homeodynamic system, and from this perspective, there is no dichotomy between the mind and body. It is the complete, harmonious functioning of the mindbody that defines health. The various sources of disruption of the energy system were carefully delineated in ancient Chinese medical texts. First, external sources of disruption were differentiated from internal ones. This differentiation was for the purpose of evaluating the patient, but does not necessarily represent exclusive categories. In fact, most often there is a great deal of overlap, with multiple sources of imbalance producing the resulting disease condition. Quite often it is difficult to differentiate sources of disharmony of the energy system, since the etiology of disease is frequently interactive and complex. The following are the external sources of imbalance:

1. **accident,** or more specifically, injuries resulting from trauma

2. **environment,** which includes weather, all forms of pollution, noise, stresses, and other more subtle factors

3. **nutrition,** including improper eating habits, or poor quality or quantity of foods

4. **microorganisms,** referring to an imbalance immunologically that results in excessive reproduction and toxic excretions

5. **exercise,** including incorrect quantity and quality

Let us now examine each of these fundamental sources of problems to understand the practical nature of the homeo-dynamic model. Accident refers to any damage or trauma to the mindbody. This may be any injury that would result in disruption of the energy system, requiring that energy be directed toward the healing of an injury. Very often the system will simply return to balance as the injury heals, but in the case of severe injury, injury to vital organs, or injuries that directly disrupt the channel, some intervention is necessary. This could take the form of helping the injury to heal by promoting circulation and lymphatic drainage and providing care for the wound, or actually in re-establishing the proper flow of energy. Accident can also include psychological trauma; a serious shock to the mindbody, such as the death of a loved one; the need for radical lifestyle changes; or even marriage. It is already clear that the concept of external/internal is artificial at best, but it does serve to differentiate pathological conditions. Injury in the area of specific energy channels or acupuncture points can often result in disruptive consequences that are often seen as separate, unconnected symptoms or produce problems months later. An injury to a finger that relates to the channel that controls digestion can often result in nausea and indigestion. Scar tissue along energy channels can also be extremely disruptive until the course of energy is restored by acupuncture or Amma therapy. This consideration is unknown to most surgeons, yet it often can provide explanation for unusual post-operative difficulties. It is important to recognize that even apparently minor traumas can have far-reaching consequences. This requires a shift in perception on the part of the health practitioner; it requires seeing the patient in a time perspective, linking past events and other aspects of the health history to help understand the patient in his or her present situation. Disease conditions are rarely specific or simple in their etiology. Even apparently simple explanations, such as "I fell and hurt my knee," should be considered in larger terms. Has the patient a history of falling accidents? Is there a propensity toward injury of a particular joint or side of the body? Is there a history of inner ear problems? As the practitioner's perspective of the patient increases, so will his understanding of the pattern of disharmony presenting itself in its present particularized symptom. On the other hand, it is equally important to recognize simple problems as such, and not create pathological conditions that aren't there. Only through careful evaluation and experience can such distinctions be made.

Environmental sources of imbalance are climatic conditions, exposure to pesticides or noxious chemicals, air and water pollution, noise pollution, or ongoing stressful living or working conditions. Included in the concept of environmental factors are energies that can effect disturbances within the mindbody. In Chinese medicine they are called the Six Pernicious Influences, or sometimes the Six Excesses, Six Evils, or Six Devils. The Six Evils are Wind, Dampness, Heat, Cold, Dryness, and Summer Heat. One way of looking at these influences is in terms of causality: seeing each of the influences as a *cause* of a disease condition. This demonstrates the idea that environmental conditions carry a particular energetic influence, and emphasizes the interactive nature of man and his environment. It is equally possible to consider disease conditions, which in Chinese medicine are called by the same names as the pernicious influences, from a non-causal perspective. Dampness and Heat also describe conditions of the internal environment, an environment that is part of a larger macrocosmos. It might be argued that the development of a particular disease condition is a result of synchrony with other energetic environments. At this point, the mindbody's propensity to respond in a particular manner is as much the cause as the external events themselves. This is the nature of the energy perspective of disease mechanisms. Certainly, other environmental factors can result in internal disharmony, such as the various forms of pollution previously mentioned. Toxic substances are ingested, breathed, or touched by people living in modern societies every day. Usually the mindbody is capable of ridding itself of such pollutants. However, excessive intake of extremely toxic substances can result in serious disruptions of the energy system. Petrochemicals, radiation, and asbestos are realities of a "civilized" society, as are food additives and preservatives. We must recognize as part of the health history the varying sensitivities individuals have to such substances, as well as factors such as strenuous exercise, which speeds the detoxification process. Contact with or ingestion of poisons is a central issue in the evaluation of nutritional patterns.

Improper nutrition is an obvious source of systemic imbalance. Foods filled with preservatives, stabilizers, colorings, and other things that are not really food require more energy of the body, to properly detoxify. Certain foods, like highly refined carbohydrates, sugar, artificial sweeteners, and some dairy products, often put great stresses on the mindbody. Some foods are carcinogenic, mucus-forming, or simply devoid of any nutritional value. The effects of poor diet can manifest themselves after many years or very quickly. All treatments directed toward rebalancing the system are effective only when accompanied by intelligent dietary changes. The mindbody is capable of dealing with a great amount of abuse, but will eventually deteriorate when the abuse is chronic. The field of nutrition is filled with controversy, and many use this as an excuse to avoid any nutritional change, but clear nutritional realities are obvious to anyone who is seriously seeking health and well-being. In general, the principle of all medicine—the avoidance of excesses—applies to nutrition. Our years of experience and experimentation at the Wholistic Health Center have produced a few basic nutritional tenets: try to eat whole, fresh, natural foods; replace refined carbohydrates with whole grains; limit the use of dairy products; and try to avoid canned or processed foods, as well as foods that are laden with preservatives or chemicals. Modern technological advances in food processing and preparation may result in changes of the energetic quality of foods in ways we do not fully understand. There is a clear energetic difference between foods baked by microwave and those baked by conventional heating methods. Unfortunately, the effects of such changes may not be understood until long after several generations have passed.

Other poisons can also be ingested in the form of over-the-counter and prescription medicines, and those, too, severely affect the harmonious balance of energy. Medication should be used with extreme caution, because the purpose of such use is symptomatic relief, and does not include an awareness of the homeodynamic balance. One of the great double-edged swords of our society has been the rapid development of the pharmaceutical industry since the 1930s. The development of antibiotics saved many lives, but the subsequent enthusiasm for the pill approach to health care has resulted in enormous abuse and excess in both the prescribing and consuming of medications. Leafing through the *Physicians' Desk Reference* should demonstrate the enormous amount of side effects and contraindications for virtually every pharmaceutical. The fundamental problem is that many people fail to recognize that medications, while often very valuable and useful, are too often applied for symptomatic relief without any consideration of the sources of the problem or the possible adverse effects of the drug. Recent research on suppressing fevers has pointed to the potential negative effects of ingesting some form of pharmaceutical every time there is an illness. Many homeopathic physicians believe that the current use of medications to suppress acute symptoms can result in an increase of chronic diseases, such as arthritis or cancer, later in a person's life. We must remember that modern medicine as we know it today is only about fifty years old. It is possible that physicians may look back a hundred years from now and wonder how we could have been so foolish.

The influence of microorganisms refers to any sort of infectious process, including viral, bacterial, fungal, or parasitic. Generally the mindbody, when in a state of homeodynamic balance, integrates and tolerates the presence of such organisms in the system. Microorganisms tend to be manifest in excessive numbers, resulting in an imbalance of the system, when the system is already tending toward imbalance. The ability of the mindbody to resist disease is a direct function of its general state of health. The more balanced the system, the greater its potential to resist disease mechanisms because of the harmonious functioning of the biological and psychological systems of the mindbody. Many believe that infectious problems are due to invasion of the system by bacteria or viruses. Usually, such microbes are in regular contact with or living within the ecosphere of the human body. The disruption of balance is more often the source of infectious disease rather than the mere presence of the microorganism. In addition, infectious problems are simply a matter of poor hygiene. Attention to cleanliness is a simple, yet powerful, method of preventative medicine. It has been said that the rapid decline of infectious disease in this century was essentially the result of better sanitation, rather than modern medicine, although antibiotics have certainly had a profound effect.

The last external source of imbalance is exercise, which also implies its opposite, proper rest. The proper quantity and quality of exercise is essential for good health. General lack of exercise results in weakness and atrophy of muscles, skeletal misalignment, poor circulation, and poor metabolism. Exercise is also the fundamental means of stimulating the lymphatic system and of cleaning the system of toxicity through perspiration. Research has shown that exercise reduces cholesterol levels and the risk of osteoporosis by stimulating an increase in bone density. Emotional well-being is also connected to proper exercise. Homeodynamic imbalance is a direct function of a lack of exercise, resulting in a wide range of health problems. The role of exercise in health care is becoming increasingly important in our sedentary society. Unfortunately, modern exercise systems are often as mechanistic as the reductionist health model. The idea of simply moving body parts, be they limbs, muscles, or heart and lungs, has become the popular conception of exercise. These approaches often do not conceive of the homeodynamic model, and miss the long-term view of health. There is insufficient attention to the quality of exercise. Exercise systems such as Hatha Yoga, T'ai Chi Chuan, and other martial arts are based upon establishing the balanced, free flow of energy in the mindbody. Such systems are important partners to mechanistic approaches because they encompass a larger view of health. They are not directed toward a cosmetic approach to health or by a narrow view aimed at the development of one particular aspect such as the cardiovascular system, as in aerobic exercise systems, but toward establishing homeodynamic balance. Certain types of movement or excessive muscular, skeletal, or cardiovascular stresses that are not carefully executed actually tend to result in imbalance and potential illness. Generally, some exercise is better than none at all, and some exercises are better than others. When an exercise program is begun, careful study and preparation are extremely important; the exercise you choose should be balanced in regard to your purposes and needs, as well as your health. A balanced lifestyle is necessary for a healthy human being.

The homeodynamic model also delineates the following factors as "internal" sources of imbalance:

1. **emotional problems,** which primarily refers to chronic emotional states

2. **physiological malfunction,** which refers to congenital defects or organ weaknesses and dysfunction

3. **musculo-skeletal misalignment,** including postural misalignment and congenital spinal problems

Emotional states, such as chronic anxiety, depression, and boredom, are given equal significance as sources of homeodynamic disruption, as are other disease processes. Such states directly disrupt the proper flow of energy, which can result in a downward emotional spiral and physical problems. A significant body of research links emotional stress with cardiovascular and respiratory problems, easily understood in terms of the "fight-flight" mechanism in animal physiology. Another interesting area of research has made dramatic links between emotional states and the autoimmune system, demonstrating increased susceptibility to infectious disease when the system is in a state of emotional imbalance. Research has been directed toward hematological analysis of immune function, in which clear immuno-suppressive effects were demonstrated where there was prolonged emotional stress.[1] An interesting study by S. V. Kasl, A. S. Evans, and J. C. Niederman in 1979 studied the incidence of mononucleosis among West Point cadets.[2] They found that the highest incidence of the disease occurred among those who shared three factors: their fathers tended to be overachievers; the cadets were highly motivated; they were doing poorly academically. There is a clear interaction between emotional states and general health. Chinese medicine makes some interesting correspondences between extreme emotional states and negative effects on the energy balance of the system. For example, anger can affect the gall bladder or liver, fear can produce problems of the kidney and bladder, and excessive joy can adversely affect the heart and small intestines. These correspondences will be discussed in a later chapter. Sometimes an energy-balancing therapy, such as acupuncture or Amma therapy, will result in a dramatic change in emotional states, but serious emotional work is also necessary for real, permanent change. Many extreme disease conditions, including cancer, have been linked to general emotional states.[3] As more research is done in these areas, there is further scientific confirmation of the truth of the homeodynamic model, a model that is at least 4,000 years old.

Physiological malfunction refers to congenital defects, weaknesses, or organ dysfunction. Studies of such problems often lead to the study of "types," that is, types of human beings who have propensities toward certain diseases. Everyone is usually a combination of types, having a pattern of innate strengths and weaknesses. Awareness of type allows an individual to pay closer attention to potential sources of health problems. The study of types has existed for thousands of years, espoused by careful observers all over the world. It is interesting to note that a landmark study of types by Dr. W. Sheldon in the United States was often maligned by his colleagues because "typing" people was "unfashionable" in a democracy, where everyone is created equal![4] It is very clear that people are not born equal, and the study of types can be extremely valuable to the health practitioner. Often the detrimental effects of physiological dysfunctions can be minimized through appropriate therapies.

Musculo-skeletal difficulties such as poor posture, skeletal misalignment, or muscular tension all tend to block the free flow of energy in the system and can result in many health problems. One of the fundamental concepts of the practice of

T'ai Chi Chuan, the Chinese exercise system, is the careful effort to maintain posture and detailed alignments of the limbs, down to the fingers. Postural alignments allow energy to flow through the system, while misalignments result in blockages that produce a wide range of dis-ease conditions. Chiropractic is founded on this concept. Energy can also be blocked by muscle tension, and postural problems can result in muscle tension or spasm, creating energy imbalances. Practices like Hatha Yoga can be extremely beneficial in helping to maintain musculo-skeletal alignment. Most ancient wholistic therapies such as Amma or acupuncture included a number of manipulative techniques to establish energy flow through the system.

Obviously these categories of sources of imbalance are not mutually exclusive, but provide a general overview of the sources of health problems. Many of these categories are clearly related and overlap each other. The wholistic approach to health is essentially "homeodynamic therapy," attempting to help the mindbody return to balance, thereby encouraging health rather than treating disease. Although wholistic practitioners will often work to alleviate symptoms, they are taken as "signs" of a larger picture—the development and maintenance of health. The various forms of homeodynamic interference clearly suggest many methods by which homeodynamic balance may be restored to the individual. For example, emotional stress could be reduced through counseling, biofeedback, exercise, Amma therapy, or acupuncture, among others. The resulting model of health care is a multimodality approach, whereby specialists in different areas, with a shared overview, approach health problems as a team, working together toward homeodynamic balance. The Amma therapist is a vital part of the wholistic team approach to health.

Endnotes   [1] See R. W. Bartrop et al., "Depressed Lymphocyte Function After Bereavement," *The Lancet*, vol. 1 (April 16, 1977), pp. 834–836; S.E. Locke et al., "Life Change Stress, Psychiatric Symptoms and Natural Killer Cell Activity," *Psychosomatic Medicine*, vol. 46 (Sept./Oct. 1984), pp. 441–453; Y. Shavit et al., "Opioid Peptides Mediate the Suppressive Effect of Stress on Natural Killer Cell Cytotoxicity," *Science*, vol. 223 (Jan., 1984), pp. 188–190.

[2] S. V. Kasi, A. S. Evans, and J. C. Niederman, "Psychosocial Risk Factors in the Development of Infectious Mononucleosis," *Psychosomatic Medicine*, vol. 41 (October, 1979), pp. 445–466.

[3] S. M. Levy, "Biobehavioral Interventions in Behavioral Medicine," *Cancer*, vol. 50 (November, 1982), pp. 1928–1935.

[4] See W. Sheldon, S. S. Stevens, W. B. Tucker, *The Varieties of Human Physique*, New York: The Hafner Publishing Company, 1970; W. Sheldon, S. S. Stevens, *The Varieties of Temperament*, New York: The Hafner Publishing Company, 1970.

CHAPTER FOUR

The Development of
the Therapist

THE evolution of an Amma therapist can be divided
into three major plateaus. At each level the practitioner appears to be treating a patient by manipulation of the soft tissues of the body in a way that is
taken to be a variant on the generally accepted techniques of
massage. Yet there is a great difference, not only between the
work of a masseuse (which is often the basis for looking at and
judging Oriental manipulative therapies by the uninitiated)
and the Amma therapist, but also among the three levels of
accomplishment of the Amma practitioner. The perspective
from which the practitioner approaches patients is considerably different, encompassing greater and greater degrees of
sensitivity to the patient as a physical, emotional, and finally
bioenergetic system. The level of technical skill, as well, that is
manifested at each level varies not only in the degree of subtlety and complexity of applicable skill and techniques, but
also in the degree of sensitivity to the flow of the bioenergy and
to the complex and subtle signals that are received.

The practice of massage by a masseuse involves various
forms of manipulation of the surface of the body, thereby
affecting the functioning of several systems, particularly the
lympathic and circulatory systems. The patient will feel generally better following a massage, and this may last for some
time. Massage helps to relieve muscular tension as well as
increase circulation and lympatic drainage. The viewpoint
from which a masseuse relates to a patient is one which takes
the physical organism to be primary. The masseuse focuses on
muscle tissue, blood, and lymphatic circulation, and seeks to

produce a state of increased circulation and muscular relaxation.

For the Amma therapist, the integrity and proper flow of energy in the physical organism is the fundamental basis of health and disease. Endogenous disease is often rooted directly in disturbance of the energy system, while exogenous disease, caused by trauma, toxins, or microorganisms, disturbs the energy system from without, limiting and inhibiting the ability of the organism to heal its physical distress. The therapist manipulates the body to engage and strengthen the body's own ability to maintain an internally regulated state of physiological and energetic balance. This uproots the underlying cause of illness, which is an imbalance of energy within the organism. The causes of these imbalances are numerous and varied, but the result of all imbalance is the same. Amma therapy, therefore, is used effectively in the treatment of both chronic and acute disorders that affect all areas of human physiology. After Amma therapy, the patient will not only feel "better," but will begin to experience a sense of vitality and well-being, and will soon discover increased awareness during normal life activities, more restful sleep, and decreased sleeping needs, as well as diminished symptoms of the primary complaint. Because Amma increases the functional energy level within the body, by reducing stress, increasing efficiency of energy production and utilization, and directly activating the energy system, the patient is able to cope more effectively with his environment and day-to-day experience.

At the highest level of accomplishment is the healing sensitive, who has evolved to the point of experiencing the highest empathy with the condition of other living beings. From a technical viewpoint it appears that a healing sensitive feels or senses the patient's energy system from the moment of even casual contact or proximity. With attention directed specifically to the patient, the physical and emotional imbalances and disturbances of the patient become known to the healing sensitive. The patient's pain, discomfort, illness—even emotional distress—are directly experienced by the healing sensitive, and inner being evolved through years of practice and intuition guides the sensitive's hands and fingers to manipulate the appropriate acupuncture points, trigger points, channels, vessels, and tissue, which almost invariably brings the patient to a state of real wellness.

One can never become a healing sensitive by studying from a book, since such an individual must function from inner being and intuition developed through years of intense and dedicated practice. Many are born with the necessary sensitivities already in place, but few are born into a situation which provides the opportunities to develop those propensities; thus, their intuitions often remain no more than good hunches and party tricks, or at best become occult clairvoyance or erratic healing abilities.

Tina Sohn is one of those very rare individuals who is a true healing sensitive—a person born with those rare abilities into a family situation where they were consciously developed. A discussion of the development of the Amma therapist, then, must include a discussion of the upbringing and training that Mrs. Sohn had as a child, for it is here that we see the physical, emotional, and mental discipline that is required to become a healing sensitive, even for those born with the capabilities inherent and partly manifest. If one is to realize the sensitivities and capabilities that are within, certain specific stages must be followed to insure the correct development of the physical body and energy body[1] as proper vehicles for the manifestation of the healing sensitivities. First, the aspirant must learn the proper technique of using the hands. The necessary physical strength and sensitivity to the body surface must be developed as the practitioner pursues the basic skills of the masseuse. Hands must become the practitioner's tools.

As the practitioner explores the personal fears and needs that are manifested within, all emotional reactions to contact with other humans must be suspended in an effort to rise above the typical human ambivalence that mars so much of human contact. Caring and compassion must take precedence over physical and emotional aversions. As physical strength, subtlety, and sensitivity develop, and the psyche is transformed, the practitioner begins to focus on the internal workings of his or her own energy system, as personal familiarity with the feel and flow of energy is prerequisite to experiencing the energy body of another. Concentration must be trained until laser-like attention can be focused upon the patient. It is only after the development of these skills that, with even greater internal discipline and effort, something far greater may become available to the evolving Amma therapist.

Mrs. Sohn was born into one of the "Eight Hundred Families," which constitute the traditional aristocracy of Korea. As a function of her birth into this family, she inherited not only the innate abilities common to the family members, but also the externally directed sense of responsibility that characterizes this royal line. All the family members have been taught to cultivate an abiding commitment to the people they serve. The women of Mrs. Sohn's family were often great healers and doctors; her father, uncles, and brothers were superior masters of the martial arts. Each individual within the family was trained in energy development and control from childhood.

Mrs. Sohn began her training when only four years old, studying disciplines akin to Hatha Yoga as well as esoteric energy development exercises. Her grandmother would execute a few Amma techniques on the child and then have the child imitate the techniques to "help grandma feel better." Thus the basic skills of the Amma therapist were inculcated into the body and hands of the child with no need for intellectual intervention. To help with the necessary physical development, she was trained as a long-distance ocean swimmer, and, by the time she had just entered adolescence, she had attained the status of champion long-distance endurance ocean swimmer. Her skill was so highly developed that she was invited to participate in the Olympic Games in the early 1950s by the Korean government.[2] Her training was so stringent that it was not sufficient simply to win after swimming twenty-five miles out and back in the Sea of Korea (or Japan, depending on the orientation of the maps used), but she was required by her coach/brother to win by several miles, and she was required to accomplish this feat without straining. After three years of competition, she did! The significance here lies not in the sport itself, but in the degree and intensity of training required to become a superior champion in any sport. In order to become a champion one must train daily for several hours; there must be a consistent and persistent effort to go beyond one's personal, physical limitations. She trained when she was well and when she was ill. She trained in heat, cold, snow, and rain. Only by training in this manner can greater and greater strength and endurance be attained. Mrs. Sohn's incredible physical strength and endurance is the result of this type of training. It must be understood that this was not a life that this child chose, but rather one that resulted from the circumstances of birth. Yet even without the driving personal desire that tends to motivate most accomplished athletes, her physical body developed into one of enormous external and internal strength.

As a result of two major shocks, the death of her father followed by the death of her older brother and first teacher within a six-month period when she was a child of twelve, she fell into a coma which lasted for thirty days. Upon awakening, the child suddenly began to see and feel strange and disturbing sensations. She "saw" her school teacher as a skeleton, and he died three months later of a consumptive disease. She "felt" pain in her kidneys while near a certain relative, and he was hospitalized with severe kidney disease several weeks later. As a result of such experiences she began to think of herself as a source of evil and to believe that she was the cause of the problems she sensed. She tried to block the experiences, and after many years had gone by in which she attempted to avoid contact and intimacy with any human being, she met the man whom she subsequently married. Under his guidance she undertook the study and discipline of her emotional nature, and her essential nature as a diagnostic sensitive and healer began to emerge. Mrs. Sohn had always believed in the Oneness of Being—that the Self within each of us is an expression of God—however, the emotional patterns and attitudes that develop in each of us as we grow into adulthood prevent us from experiencing the nature of this truth. Her belief became a living reality for her through the esoteric psychological work taught and directed by her husband and teacher, Robert Sohn.

The emotional nature of each man or woman is built on desire, which in turn breeds, anger, fear, jealousy, and other emotions which serve only to isolate us from the conscious experiencing of the reality of our own inner world, the world around us, and the people with whom we interact and relate. She was not different. But by deep study, sincere self-observation, and unmerciful self-analysis, she looked directly at the nature of these emotional states and how they were the driving forces in her life (as they are in virtually all lives). She was able to harness the energy that was previously wasted in pointless emotionality, and use the energy to develop herself. Through years of self-study and internal psychological discipline and direction, she was transformed into an extraordinary woman with acute sensitivities and understanding. This understanding allows her to be a true diagnostic sensitive. It guides her, through her highly developed and disciplined skills as a therapist, to perceive the ailment and how to heal it, and often to become the medium, herself, for healing. That understanding is an inner connection to the reality of the Nature of the Being of Man; the Reality of the Oneness of Being; and the inter-relationship of all humans and creatures through the Universal Self. Knowing and feeling herself to be more than a material body, the master Amma therapist is enlivened by inner Understanding, and is thus a truly unique individual. To touch and grow into what Mrs. Sohn has become, a therapist must take on and practice the discipline of mind and body that she practiced to its ultimate end.

The development of a therapist begins with training the physical body with at least a twofold purpose. Physical strength is necessary for an Amma therapist just as it is for a masseuse; in fact, since Amma encompasses all the techniques of Shiatsu, Rolfing, and Tui Na, as well as what is commonly misnamed acupressure, and many additional skills of body manipulation, the Amma practitioner must be equal to any professional athlete in strength and stamina. The training is also designed to produce direct experiential understanding of the body's internal functioning. There is no better way to study living anatomy than to seek to understand your own body. Several techniques are used to develop this combined academic and experiential knowledge of the human organism. Included among these are T'ai Chi Chuan and Hatha Yoga.

Hatha Yoga is a system of relaxed exercise in which various muscle groups are stretched or strengthened by developing and maintaining specific postures for short time periods. Once the posture is accomplished, the practitioner focuses attention on the specific area of the body under tension, concentrates on the muscles and tendons that are being used, and practices intentional relaxation of those tensed muscles and tendons. By directing attention to the muscle groups, and attempting conscious control of their responses, an uncommon awareness of the location and function of the various muscles is developed. (People involved in the sport of bodybuilding have some degree of this awareness, and in many cases, Amma practitioners are advised and guided in necessary and appropriate resistance training exercises). Muscular strength and coordination are produced. Flexibility, balance, and concentration are developed. All of these physical qualities are essential for one who will be engaged in the vigorous and rigorous activity of the application of Amma therapy. When practiced by one who is studying or has studied anatomy and myology, Hatha Yoga becomes a living experience of what was previously only classroom study. It is only through this proper effort of mind and body that a real understanding of the capabilities and functioning of the human body can be attained.

Through consistent and correct practice, the internal processes of the body also become part of the cognitive awareness of the practitioner. Since controlled breathing is part of the Hatha Yoga practice, the respiratory system and the musculature involved in respiration can be contacted and their mechanisms developed toward optimum functioning. Processes involved in digestion and elimination can be sensed, aided, and, with advanced practice, controlled. With the modern recognition that stress is an important component of poor circulation, it becomes obvious that the direction of attention to relaxation of the musculature and balanced and controlled breathing can be a significant factor in the promotion of a healthy circulatory system. Correct posture and spinal alignment, and the effects of posture on the physical processes, become part of the awareness. The postures of Hatha Yoga massage the inner organs, reducing fat and increasing muscle tone in these hard-to-reach areas. All of these benefits lead to a healthier and more physically fit practitioner. Physical health should be a requisite for any person preparing to treat the ailments of another.

Most humans have little or no awareness of the three-dimensional, living, physical body. In fact, we tend to sense ourselves as a two-dimensional surface that primarily encompasses only our face and upper chest. The practice of Hatha Yoga expands the awareness to include the internal as well as the surface aspects of the physical body. This internal awareness is essential for the proper development of an Amma therapist. It can and should be the basis of the evolution of a much greater understanding of the physical difficulties that patients encounter in both stress and illness. This results in an easier and clearer understanding of the means that must be used to help patients. You know yourself as a physical body, and you can therefore know your patient's physical experiences more fully.

We must remember, however, that Amma therapy is far more than a simple massage that affects the physical body. Amma's major concern is the manipulation and harmonization of the energy system and its profound effects on the physical body. It is directed at the production of the homeodynamic state. There is, of course, transmission of energy from the practitioner to the patient, and this transmission is amplified by the techniques of Amma and their direct effect on the energy body. The physical condition and psychological and emotional energies of the practitioner have effects upon the concomitant areas in the patient. This accounts for the need for physical, psychological, and emotional development of the therapist. During the administration of Amma therapy by a physically, psychologically, and emotionally developed therapist, powerful effects upon the three-part nature of the patient can be accomplished. In order to bring such effects to their maximum potential, given the limits imposed by the prior deterioration of each patient, the practitioner of Amma therapy must learn to directly experience his or her own energy body as well as the energy body of the patient. Subsequent control of the energy systems of both the practitioner and the patient leads to the very advanced, sometimes profound, results clearly seen and experienced in the work of Mrs. Sohn and other, albeit rare, healing sensitives.

To facilitate the goal of becoming a master Amma therapist, T'ai Chi Chuan, a Taoist form of exercise and active meditation, is studied for the development of the level of awareness and for control of one's own energy system. The practice of T'ai Chi Chuan is the effort to create a mind-to-energy-to-physical-body pathway—that is, to establish mind control over the energy so that the energy may properly control and move the body. As a result of the concentration and practice of subtle awareness required to master T'ai Chi Chuan, the movement of energy becomes a cognitive experience for the practitioner. The practice of T'ai Chi Chuan, under appropriate conditions of instruction and effort, can ultimately lead the Amma therapist to a point of direct conscious experience of energy deficiencies and excesses, as they exist in the physical body of the patient, and thereby produce effects that are far more substantial than when the practitioner works in the dark.

Although the development of physical strength and control and energy awareness and control are fundamental to the art of Amma therapy, another aspect of development is of equal or even greater significance—work on one's own emotional nature. In order to see and feel another's physical and emotional experiences, great effort must be made to see and to feel one's own emotional experiences. Without this there can be no clarity of vision. A major part of the human experience is the emotional component. Our experience of the world around us, the people with whom we communicate, and our relationships to our spouses, our families, our jobs, and our living situations is colored by our inner, emotional experience. There is a direct relationship between our emotional states and the condition of our physical body. A major component of physical disease is very often emotional experience. In order to treat disease we must see its emotional side. We must see the way others experience their world, and we must see the various ways in which their perspectives can be expanded in order to cope more effectively with themselves and their environment. There is no way to do this without knowing oneself fully. Thus, a fundamental part of becoming a therapist is the evolution of self-awareness of the three levels: physical body, energy body, and psychological body. By studying our inner, psychological nature, we can observe how we actually see the world (which is often quite different from what we believe it is), our personal difficulties, and, ultimately, the ways to expand and change our perspectives in order to cope more effectively with ourselves and our environment. It is necessary to have the help of another so that we can learn to see what we are as emotional beings. Just as we need teachers to help us train our physical and energy bodies, we need a teacher to help us gain an objective understanding of our emotional world. Through this objective direction we can learn to deal with those aspects of our inner world which are psychologically painful and which prevent us from seeing others clearly. The discipline of our emotional nature is the primary means of energy conservation, and since an Amma therapist must work directly with the energy of a patient, the work on inner awareness becomes one of the most important and basic efforts of the aspiring master Amma therapist.

To a true health professional, concern for the well-being of patients is absolutely necessary, and must be cultivated far beyond the normal levels of human concern. However, we cannot create a new emotional experience within, without first seeing what is already present in our emotional environments. We must be acutely aware of ourselves, our requirements of our patients, our attachments to being treated with respect or with equality, or our responses to touching another human being physically and psychologically. In the process of evaluating and treating patients, we must put aside the personality responses to others that are a function of typical emotional relationships. A therapist must develop the skill of concern without attachment. As a teacher and healer, the Amma practitioner must maintain a certain objectivity that is easily lost when common friendship is cultivated. A therapist must understand the difficulties experienced by patients. There is no place in the practitioner-patient relationship for disdain, condemnation, or any other negative emotion. A patient must be guided with understanding and a valuation for the level of health that may be attained through the joint efforts of the practitioner-patient team. Yet we cannot force patients to make efforts. We can suggest, we can encourage, we can even motivate with stronger means if the circumstances require it and if the therapist can maintain objectivity. We must do this out of our own responsibility to our patients. Treating another human being must never be taken lightly. The practitioner must always remember that another person's health, well-being, quality of life, and perhaps quantity of life has been entrusted to him. This must be considered and felt with great seriousness and must never be forgotten.

One additional area must be discussed, and although it may seem obvious, experience has shown us that a certain remnant of the lower aspects of New Age morality has clouded this issue for many of the practitioners of various massage styles. Personal cleanliness is absolutely necessary. Poor hygiene is one of the primary contributing factors in ill health and disease. In order to maintain health one must keep one's body clean, internally as well as externally. This includes daily showering or bathing, washing your hair, brushing your teeth, cleansing your hands and nails, washing your genitals and rectum, and washing internally if you are a female. For the comfort of both the practitioner and the patient, your clothing must be clean and free of unpleasant odors.

Since many aspects of health are correlated to diet and bowel habits, it is important to keep your digestive system functioning effectively for both your personal nutrition and the elimination of waste. Your diet should consist of unprocessed whole grains, fresh fruits and vegetables, fish, poultry, and lean meat. Processed foods should be avoided; dairy food, salt, and sugar should be extremely limited. Foods that contain chemical additives and preservatives should be avoided. Clean water should be part of your diet, both in drinking and for use in cooking. Distilled water or spring water is preferable to tap water in most areas of the United States. In general, this is the same type of diet that would be recommended to your patients—a natural, whole foods diet. By adopting this diet, you can accomplish two things. First, you will become healthier, clearer, and more energetic. Second, you will be able to understand any difficulties that your patients may have in adopting this type of diet. For both reasons you will be better able to understand your patient and will therefore be of greater help in your ministrations.

To become a being capable of sensing and manipulating the energies of another, and to be able to feel another's inner physical and emotional experience, is to embark on a journey which develops much more than a simple art of treatment. There is a spiritual aspect of our being that lies hidden beneath our desires and personality experiences of pleasure and pain. A master Amma therapist is one who is in full inner accord with that spiritual existence, who knows the fullness of Being. To begin to touch this understanding, attachment to the surface must be seen and experienced for what it is in its limited and pointless nature. Through consistent effort to uncover and nurture the deeper nature of humankind, to free yourself from the emptiness of selfish existence and touch the deeper reality you share with the rest of nature, the power to understand the suffering of others and the knowledge of how best to alleviate that suffering become yours. In this very process you gain health, strength, wisdom, freedom, and joy. It is from this deep, inner place that a true healer can be born.

Endnotes

[1] Eastern cultures have known for thousands of years that a being is more than a mere physical body. This truth is fundamental to all spiritual teachings throughout the ages, the study and practice of acupuncture, and the advanced forms of the martial arts. That which enlivens the physical body is a body of energy: a system complete within itself, having clearly defined patterns of flow. We refer to this energy system as the energy body.

[2] Her family would not allow her to do this. She also trained, in what she believed was secrecy, in the complex Korean Drum Dance and in theatrical singing, but her family intervened when she planned to perform. They could accept any study for self-improvement and development, but never for performance.

PART TWO

The Principles

————————————

CHAPTER FIVE

Introduction to Basic Oriental Anatomy and Physiology

Primary Distinctions between Western and Oriental Viewpoints

FOREWORD The following discussion of the basic principles of Chinese medical theory is only a preliminary attempt to introduce the apparently exotic basis of this medical science. Subsequent books in this series will attempt to explain the concepts surrounding diagnosis and treatment patterns so that they can become the basis of a realistic appraisal and evaluation of the patient. For now, we wish to acquaint the first-time student of Chinese medicine with the proper philosophical basis for beginning to understand the purpose and real nature of the art of Amma therapy. Those whose knowledge exceeds such entry-level information may skip the following sections, although some fresh views may appear for those interested in skimming through what follows. It is necessary to reorient the thinking process so that the functional and not the structural elements of the diagnosis become the basis of the treatment pattern to follow. To facilitate an awareness of this difference, we have chosen to capitalize many words which would not ordinarily be capitalized, hoping to remind the reader of the extraordinary usages being implied. We do this (a practice which has become common in English writings on Oriental medicine) to remind the reader to distinguish the more intangible, energetic meaning of the terms as used in Chinese medicine from the very concrete and palpable items of the Western tradition. Oriental diagnosis and therapy is concerned with the dynamic balance of the interactive forces of the individual cosmos of each human. Structure may be considered to the extent that it is clearly structural defect that is the basis of the disease condition; however, the following brief story from my own experience with acupuncture illustrates the real functional concern of Chinese medicine as opposed to the allopathic physician's concern for structure.

Several years ago a young woman of twenty-five who had been deaf in the right ear since the age of four as a result of childhood otitis media asked to be treated with acupuncture, since she had read that deafness was being cured in China by acupuncture. After twenty treatments, the hearing in her deaf right ear was totally restored. She could cover the left ear and hear perfectly, including whispers; she could carry on a telephone conversation with the telephone held against the previously deaf ear; and she could no longer sleep blissfully through storms and sirens even if her "deaf" ear was exposed while the other ear was buried in a pillow. Her life became absolutely normal. She went to the ear specialist who was amazed at the results and asked to do a test on the right auditory nerve. The examination showed that the nerve was dead and could not be conducting the sounds that she heard. The allopathic physician then announced solemnly that *the acupuncture had not worked* and that the young woman was *still deaf in the right ear.* Thus, his concern lay with the functionless structure, while our concern, and that of the patient, who contended that she was no longer deaf, was with function, even this apparently structureless function which constituted this young woman's hearing.[1]

As is clear from the above story, the Chinese traditional physician has a view of the problem which is more akin to that of the patient. When the patient has pain, the Amma therapist, like the Chinese traditional physician, should seek the cause of the pain in the imbalance of Yin and Yang, and, if there are indeed structural disturbances, to be aware that, although the repair of structure may relieve the problem, it also may not. What is apparently irreparable by traditional Western means, may be sometimes rather easily resolved by traditional Oriental means, and many functional repairs can be made in spite of remaining structural disturbance, as is so clearly illustrated in the deaf young woman's recovery. One more small example may suffice. Herpes zoster is a disease that often defies the traditional allopathic medical treatment. Although medications will often relieve the structural symptoms of the disease, i.e., stop the itching and the blister-like red and running pustules that form, it will often leave the patient with the sometimes excruciating problem of postherpetic pain syndrome. Acupuncture will often relieve both the physical (structural) symptoms and the pain. Sometimes the pain will go long before the skin has healed, and in most cases both acupuncture and Amma therapy can relieve the terrible post-herpetic pain that is the worst aspect of herpes zoster, and undoubtedly beyond the scope of allopathic treatments in almost all cases.

FUNCTIONAL VS. STRUCTURAL VIEWPOINT

The interesting and very important difference between the views of the Western and Oriental health practitioner—the dichotomy between the significance given to form and function—has deep and primary implications. This distinction defines the entry point and primary direction of the whole of the theoretical and practical process of the health care system. While the Western practitioner is very conscious of form, and its concomitant relationship to structure, his Oriental counterpart is primarily concerned with function. This difference is most markedly obvious in the study of the Oriental concept of the Organs. Students of Western anatomy and physiology are introduced to detailed studies of the structures of the major systems and of the important organs of the body: the osseous system, the nervous system, the vascular system, the lymphatic system, the genitourinary system, the endothelial-reticular system, the gastrointestinal system, the tegumentary system, the pulmonary system, the organs of special sense, and others as well. All are studied in very great detail, and their functions are directly tied to their individual structures and to structural relationships. Function is thus defined in terms of structure. While Western anatomy and physiology are concerned with the physical body in its most concrete form, Oriental healing arts have deeper concerns related to the underlying and sustaining body of energy which enlivens the physical form. Thus, our concern is not with the structure and structure-related functions of the physical body, but with the energy and functionally related structures. For example, from the Western medical perspective, the anatomy of the spleen is highly evolved, providing the minutest detail of the tissue structure and its differentiation, careful analysis of the organ's ennervation, detailed knowledge of its vascularization, and specific details of its size, shape, placement, support, position in relation to other organs, attachments, and every other imaginable physical detail. However, there is very little knowledge, and not a great deal of conjecture, as to its function. And it is removed with impunity by surgeons. Of course, it can be injured beyond repair, but the concept of why it ought to be repaired is missing. The pancreas is known in the same minute detail as the spleen, and its function is known to some degree—it is seen as necessary to supplement the secretions of the pancreas as soon as the blood sugar balance becomes consistently impaired—however, the ability to repair that function is not ever considered.

Oriental medical science, on the other hand, gives virtually no description of the spleen or the pancreas. There are some simple drawings made on occasion by curious physicians, and these tend to show the spleen as a roundish organ in the left hypochondriac region with a long tail reaching almost to the liver. This tail is obviously the pancreas, since there is no knowledge of the pancreas as a separate organ. The functions of the pancreas are considered to be part of the functional orb of the Spleen. The Spleen is specified as the controller of the digestive function. It harbors Shen, or the Human Spirit. It communicates with the Lung (in that they share the same type of energy differentiation, which will be explained later), and enters into disease syndromes involving many other organs. It couples with the Stomach (the concept of coupled channels and organs will be discussed), and together they constitute the Middle Warmer, wherein the process of digestion is accomplished. Its energy is the Great Yin, and therefore it is the very beginning of the cycle of life, which begins with the ingestion of Air into the Lung and the ingestion of food into the digestive tract of the Stomach and Intestines. Since the Spleen is the controller of the total function, it regulates, balances, and nourishes, but does not directly digest the food.

This clear distinction between the two systems shows that they are indeed complementary and not antagonistic, as many in both communities seem to feel. Dr. Manfred Porket takes great pains to show this truth in the introduction to his second book, *The Essential of Chinese Diagnostics*, where he develops the complementary nature of the Chinese synthetic as opposed to the Western analytic approach. I highly recommend that introduction for a further study of this important issue.[2]

Basic Concepts Underlying the Chinese Medical Model

YIN/YANG   The Chinese base their entire medical system on the idea of a polarity of forces which actively change throughout the day, season, and lifetime, but which maintain a certain balance, which we have named the homeodynamic balance (see Chapter 3), and this homeodynamic balance is the basis of the function of the whole mechanism. The basic manifestations of these forces as polarities are called Yin and Yang. The concept of antagonistic forces as mutually supportive is not alien to Western medical thought, and can be seen superficially in the antagonistic muscle pairs (the extensors and flexors which allow us to move) and more deeply in the complex chemical and neurological activities of the body in which inhibition and stimulation are constantly at play to maintain the homeodynamic condition which is the organism's most stable state.

Although there are a number of classic examples of Yin/Yang pairings—such as the very basic Yang is male and Yin is female—these concepts are rooted in a cultural viewpoint which allowed easy understanding of what is now a complex, derivative concept. I shall avoid controversy and list only the examples that seem rather clear and are used diagnostically in the health field. In future works the more complex concepts will be addressed.

Yang is Heaven, the Sun, Bright, External, Hollow, tends to float, Energy. Yin is Earth, the Moon, Dark, Internal, Solid, tends to sink, Matter. Yet, the energy of Heaven which is Yang moves down to become Yin, and the Energy which is Yin moves up to become Yang. The value of the concepts is primarily in the pattern differentiation that defines the basic diagnostic techniques of Oriental medicine. The Amma therapist must understand the Eight Principles which are the cornerstone of Chinese diagnosis. Disease is classified first into some pattern of the Eight Principles: Yang or Yin, Hot or Cold, External or Internal, Excess or Deficient. A Hot disease of Yang Organs of external origin and showing Excess is clearly a Yang disease, but an Excess Cold disease of a Yang Organ of internal origin is clearly mixed Yin and Yang. There are no absolutes, only relative degrees of relativity.

Oriental medical science further divides these two basic antagonistic/supportive forces of Yin and Yang, first into the six transitory stages of Yin and Yang, and then into the Five

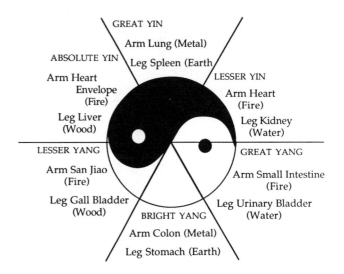

GREAT YIN
Arm Lung (Metal)
ABSOLUTE YIN   Leg Spleen (Earth)
Arm Heart   LESSER YIN
Envelope   Arm Heart
(Fire)   (Fire)
Leg Liver   Leg Kidney
(Wood)   (Water)
LESSER YANG   GREAT YANG
Arm San Jiao   Arm Small Intestine
(Fire)   (Fire)
Leg Gall Bladder   Leg Urinary Bladder
(Wood)   (Water)
BRIGHT YANG
Arm Colon (Metal)
Leg Stomach (Earth)

Figure 1

Phases or Relative Motions (energies) commonly called the Five Elements. The six stages of the manifestation of Yin and Yang are usually referred to by American acupuncturists as the Six Chiao (pronounced "jow"). They can best be shown in their graphic or symbolic representations in the modified classical Yin/Yang diagram (see Figure 1).

Sometimes charts show the Absolute Yin (also translated Diminishing Yin) as the middle Yin stage. It will become obvious with further explanation that this is indeed the true pattern. The cycle of activity begins in the quiescence of the Great Yin, which then swells into the Absolute Yin. Absolute Yin, reaching the ultimate peak of Yin, turns rapidly into its opposite and becomes the Lesser Yang.[3] The Lesser Yang grows into the Bright Yang, and then swells into the Great Yang, and reaching the ultimate peak of Yang, turns rapidly into its opposite and becomes the Lesser Yin. Yin and Yang flow into each other and turn into each other. They are mutually supportive yet are in constant conflict.

In this discussion, and more acutely in the discussion that follows, you will notice that more than one phrase or term is used to describe the same concept. This results from the fact that the Chinese medical concepts are often very different in meaning from their directly translated English counterparts.

THE PATTERN OF
THE FIVE RELATIVE
PHASES

The Five Relative Phases are commonly called the Five Elements. This caused an early negative response from many Western health professionals and those who thought themselves enlightened in modern scientific terms and knew that there were, indeed, more than ninety elements. Just as the ancient Greeks, in their philosophical search for the nature of the "underlying substance," used the metaphors of major natural phenomena to name energies, the Chinese and the East Indians used similar conceptualizations to express the general relative forces at play. They continued to use the same terms to describe similar forces at play in much more specific areas. Thus, the Five Relative Phases became the basis of much of the diagnostics of Chinese medicine. The Five Phases are, proceeding from most Yang to most Yin: Fire, Water, Wood, Earth, and Metal. These Five Phases were used as categories for the classification of virtually all natural phenomena, and as a whole this classification system is termed the "correspondences." These correspondences are clearly stated in the Chinese medical literature and are part of the backbone of the diagnostic art. In each major area of concern, factors are generally organized into groups of five. Sometimes there is a real correspondence; sometimes they are forced for philosophical continuity. Clinical experience is the best teacher of what is real.

We include a chart showing several of the important correspondences for use in diagnostics (see Table 1).

Although various combinations of the Five Elemental Phases are possible, two have great significance to the practitioner of Oriental medicine. Just as Yin and Yang are in a combined antagonistic/supportive relationship, the Five Phases also show the same "balanced stress" in the Cycles of Creation (support) and Destruction (control).

In Figure 2, the Cycles of Creation and Destruction are shown graphically. The outer cycle is the Creation Cycle; the inner cycle (the five-pointed star) is the Control Cycle. The

TABLE 1

Relative Phase	Yin Viscera	Yang Bowels	Sense Organ	Tissue	Color	Emotion	Season	Climate
FIRE	Heart	Small Intestine	Tongue	Blood Vessels	Red	Joy	Summer	Heat
EARTH	Spleen	Stomach	Mouth	Flesh	Yellow	Contemplation	Late Summer	Damp
METAL	Lung	Colon	Nose	Skin/Hair	Ashen (white)	Sadness	Autumn	Dryness
WATER	Kidney	Urinary Bladder	Ear	Bones	Black	Fear	Winter	Cold
WOOD	Liver	Gall Bladder	Eye	Tendons	Green	Anger	Spring	Wind

pattern of relationship is based on the law called Mother/Son, in which Fire is the Mother of Earth and Earth is the Son of Fire, Earth is the Mother of Metal and Metal is the Son of Earth. Mother supports Son, while the Mother of the Mother controls the Son. If the Mother is weak, it does not feed the Son and weakens the Son in turn. If the Son becomes Excess, it can draw excessively on the Mother, injuring the Mother. In the control cycle there can be overcontrol, or an unnatural reversal in which the controlled injures the controller. The complex effects of this pattern constitute one of the most important diagnostic and treatment techniques of Chinese medicine.

The true wisdom of the basic theory is illustrated by Figure 2. Note the controlling function of the Wood Liver and Gall Bladder over the Earth Stomach and Spleen. If we simply think of the angry and stressful business man who develops ulcers and finds it difficult to digest fatty foods, we can easily see how the Chinese functional model clearly explains the problem, which only recently became slightly less opaque to the structurally oriented physician.[4] Excess anger is an increase of Liver Fire (there is Fire in the Liver and in the Kidney as well, but explanations of such complexities are better left to a later text), and, because of the coupled relationship between the two, causes overactivation of Liver Wood. It generally follows that there is overcontrol of Earth by Wood. This injures the Spleen (disturbing the whole digestive process), and further causes the stomach to act inefficiently and eat into its own lining, causing an ulcer. The excess of the Gall Bladder makes its digestive function highly inefficient, and the resulting condition is as indicated above. The Amma therapist must treat the

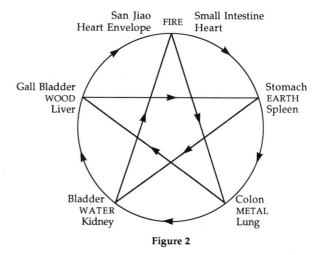

Figure 2

Liver and Gall Bladder to calm and correct their function, while treating the Stomach and Spleen to support and assist them. Stress management and dietary recommendations would, of course, be appropriate. Thus it can be seen, if only in a rudimentary fashion, that the Five Phases play a very important role in the differential diagnosis of the advanced Amma therapist.

QI, BLOOD, AND FLUIDS

One of the most fundamental ideas in the Chinese medical model, is the concept of *qi* (pronounced "chee"), which, although translated as "energy" for a long time, has not been understood by the Western practitioner in a real and dynamic sense. A sad realization is that much New Age usage of the word "energy" is as an abstract idea without direct experiential relationship to the concept. *Qi*, in its many manifestations, is a real and concrete experience for those who seek to realize its presence. In its simplest, conceptual form, *qi* is expressed in the phrases "I have a lot of energy today," and its negative counterpart, "I feel really low on energy, I can't seem to think straight, get anything right, or finish my work." But for the practitioner of Amma and other Chinese medical arts, *qi* becomes a large and important variety of different manifestations. Yin and Yang are the great dichotomies of *qi*. The Six Chiao are forms that it takes, as well as the Five Relative Phases. However, these are general and abstract concepts, and the *qi* becomes more specific when we begin to look at the organ complex and the absorption and creation of various forms of the active *qi* of the body. We will give a general description of the absorption and creation of *qi*, and this will be reiterated with some more detail in the brief discussion of the orbs of influence of the organs and the channels.

Before birth the child is sustained by the *qi* of the mother, and a very precious substance is created and passed on to the child in the procreation/birth process. This is the Prenatal Qi called the Qi of Prior Heaven (*hsien-tien qi*). *Hsien-tien qi* can be conceived as the hereditary constitutional potential of the body. In its kinetic aspect, it is known to circulate in the channels and to enter into all transforming processes. It is then called Yuan Qi, or the Active Essence of the Kidney. This substance is stored in the Kidney and carried by the Leg Lesser Yin Channel, as well as by the Eight Extra Channels. This energy motivates or activates the flow of *qi* in the channels, and it acts as the catalyst for all the processes of energy creation through digestion as well as for the cycle of energy usage and generation in the organs.

After birth the child breathes, and ingests not only the oxygen known so well in the Western world, but also the Qi of Air. As the child eats or drinks its first food, the Stomach and the Spleen act to extract that substance called Ku Qi, or the Qi of Grain, which is transmitted by the Spleen to the Lung. Here the two forms of *qi* are combined, influenced by the catalytic action of Yuan Qi, the kinetic aspect of Prenatal Qi, to form the Nutrient Qi which flows in the channels. See p. 56 for a more complete explanation of this process.

Now, as the *qi* flows through the organ cycle, each organ uses what is necessary for its functions and adds to the general flow, and some of the organs generate Defensive Qi, which flows in the Tendino-Muscle channels and in the Cutaneous Regions. It is believed that the Defensive Qi may flow in the Divergent channels as well. However, the Divergent channels will not be explored in this text.

In addition to the work of transforming and transporting *qi*, the digestive function is concerned with the creation of two additional substances. After the *qi* has been extracted by the Spleen, and the remaining substance is passed to the small intestine, another process of separation occurs, in which the pure fluids are separated from the impure substances. These fluids are then circulated in a number of differentiations such as serous fluid, saliva, sweat, or synovial fluids. Some of the pure fluid is combined with *qi* to produce the substance called Blood, which only in part refers to blood as it is known in the West. In the Chinese view, one refined form of Blood flows in the channels with the *qi* (as, of course, *qi* flows with the more material aspect of Blood in the blood vessels). Blood is a complex substance, which changes as it moves through the system, and partakes both of material and energetic qualities. Blood is the Yin of the Heart, and Fire is the Yang of the Heart. It could be looked at as the most Yin, or palpable, part of the *qi*. Many of the disease syndromes or patterns are considered conditions of the *qi* or Blood, and the relation of these two is not unlike the relations between the Yin/Yang pairs of the channels or the Eight Principles. This will be discussed in a later text as specifically related to Amma therapy. General discussions of the topic are available in many acupuncture texts.

Qi, Blood, and fluids will be discussed in somewhat more detail at the end of the next section.

Oriental Physiology: the Functional Orbs of the Bowels and Viscera

Oriental medicine notes the existence of ten or eleven organs, one or two functions, and a number of lesser organs which are hardly mentioned except in the context of their dysfunctions. The Six Yin Viscera, or "organs of constant physiology," or "solid organs," are the Lung, Spleen, Heart, Kidney, Envelope of the Heart, and Liver. The Six Yang Bowels, or "organs of intermittent physiology," or "hollow organs," are the Colon, Stomach, Small Intestine, Urinary Bladder, San Jiao (Three Burning Spaces), and Gall Bladder. There are minor organs such as the brain which do not enter into the primary and secondary energy cycles, and are therefore given limited consideration. The uterus is considered significant in that it is the place of arising of certain extra channels. The organs of special sense are connected to the orbs of influence of the Bowels and Viscera. "Orb," in this context, refers to the sphere of influence, or area over which influence is exercised, of the Bowels and Viscera. Other important tissue groups are also related to the control or influence of certain Bowels and Viscera. As we discuss the Organs it will become apparent that we are not discussing the Western physical structures. The structures are indeed noted and are even outlined in the charts of the pathways of the channels. But, as previously discussed, the function is the focus of interest, and the surgical removal of an organ does not remove the function, although it definitely hinders that function. We will take each of the major Viscera/Bowels in turn, discussing them as Yin/Yang pairs as they are coupled in their pertaining channels, and describing their function and sphere of influence within the physical body.

LUNGS AND COLON   The Lung[5] is often referenced in Chinese medical literature as the Delicate Organ because it is the first of the organs to be injured by negative substances or energies (called Evil qi in Chinese medicine) entering with air. Its pertaining sense organ is the nose. It is in control of qi and air and has the property of dispersing and descending; it therefore spreads qi, Blood, and Vital Fluids throughout the body and causes air and qi to descend. It also regulates water passages. Its dispersing function causes the excretion of sweat, thereby helping regulate temperature and detoxification, while its descending function causes fluids to pass down to the Kidney to be excreted as urine, again aiding in detoxification and basic elimination. The

Lung dominates the skin and hair, disperses the nutritive energy to the total body surface, and, through the control of Wei (defensive) Qi, opens and closes the pores, and is generally in charge of the first lines of defense of the organism. Since the Lung is involved with the process of bringing *qi* and air into the body and dispersing them, and since the nose is the "gateway" of *qi* and air, the health of the Lung will be reflected in conditions of the nose and para-nasal sinuses.

The Colon is in charge of the salvage of water from the impure matter passed on to it by the Small Intestine. Like its Yin counterpart, it is involved in water metabolism. It is interesting to note here that the functions of the more superficial Yang organs are described in more concrete terms, and therefore are closer to the conceptions of the Western trained health professional.

The Lung and Colon have the following diagnostically significant Five Phase correspondences as they are assigned to the Metal Phase: the season of autumn, the climatic condition of dry, the color white, the melancholy emotion, the pungent taste, and the sound of crying or sobbing.

SPLEEN AND STOMACH

Although the function of the Spleen was discussed above, we shall elaborate on that discussion here. The Spleen controls digestion while the Stomach receives the substances to be digested. Thus the Spleen is responsible for the transformation and transportation of Nutrient Qi. It produces Blood and keeps the Blood in the vessels. It opens into the mouth and controls the limbs and the flesh.

The Stomach receives food, and, under the control of the Spleen, separates the Nutrient Qi from the substance of food. The Spleen transports the Nutrient Qi up to the Lung for further processing, while the Stomach moves the substance down to the Small Intestine for continued digestion and assimilation. The Spleen likes dry, but easily can become excessively damp, creating diarrhea. The Spleen Qi, also called Middle Qi, is responsible for keeping the organs in their places; therefore, when the Spleen is healthy there will not be any prolapses of the stomach, bladder, or rectum. The Spleen is also responsible for keeping the blood circulating in the vessels. Thus unexplained bleeding as well as hemorrhaging in the skin, so common in diabetes, is a failure of the Spleen function.[6] It is also said in the classics that the Spleen dominates the muscles, and that the Spleen's proper control of transportation and transformation of nutrients determines their density and strength.

The Spleen has been indicated as the controller of the digestive functions. This is not as alien to the Western view as it may at first seem. Studies in dogs, for example, have shown that the spleen holds extra quantities of blood, and that this extra blood is released as soon as the digestive process is stimulated. Although Chinese traditional medicine did not have any specific knowledge of the pancreas, the function of the pancreas, in relation to sugar balance, was known to be controlled by the Spleen. Again the work of Dr. Reinhold Voll has shown that the right side Leg Great Yin Spleen Channel acts as if it were a Great Yin Pancreas Channel, and certain points on the foot of the right side Leg Great Yin show very specific effects on certain tissue and functions of the pancreas.[7] The Spleen is said to harbor *shen* or the human spirit (this is not to be confused with the *name* of the Kidney in Chinese, which is also *shen*).

The Spleen and Stomach have the following diagnostically significant Five Phase correspondences as they are assigned to the Earth Phase: the later part of the summer season, and the phenomenon called "Indian Summer," the climatic condition of damp (although the Spleen tends toward dryness), the color yellow, the pensive emotion, the sweet taste, and the sound of singing.

The pertaining channels of the two Viscera/Organ pairs just described constitute the first four channels of the primary energy cycle. The Great Yin of the Lung and Spleen surround the Bright Yang of the Colon and Stomach, and the energy manifests most actively in the Lung from 3 to 5 A.M., in the Colon from 5 to 7 A.M., in the Stomach from 7 to 9 A.M., and in the Spleen from 9 to 11 A.M. Here we begin to see the basis for the lifestyles of yogis, Buddhist monks, and others. One should awaken at 3 A.M. and do breathing exercises and postures until the day's bowel movement sometime between 6 and 7 A.M. The day's meal should be taken preferably before 9 A.M., and one should never eat after 11 A.M. It is obvious that when the Lung Qi is at its strongest, it will be most efficient in absorbing oxygen and the Qi of Air necessary for the creation of the body's need for various forms of *qi*. It is also a time for meditative breathing in the calm of the morning, when the purity of the *qi* in the air and the strength of the *qi* of the Lungs can interact to produce the Ancestral Qi which resides in the Conception channel. It is a time when the whole process of conversion of *qi* into the theoretically limited Prenatal Qi of the Kidney can indeed be accomplished. This, of course, is the point of the lives of the monks and yogis of whom we speak.

HEART AND SMALL
INTESTINE

The Heart controls the blood vessels and houses the mind. It opens into the tongue, and the tongue is used extensively in diagnosis, particularly to indicate Heart-related problems. The condition of the Heart is reflected in the face. "The Heart controls the blood vessels" really means that the Heart is responsible for the movement of the Blood in the vessels.[8] The Sovereign Fire of the system is in the Heart, and the Fire is the Yang of the Heart. The Blood is the Yin of the Heart. "The Heart stores the Spirit" means that the Heart is involved with all mental activities such as thought, memory, or sleep. The Spirit of the Heart and the Essence of the Kidney together constitute the consciousness of the organism.

The Small Intestine separates waste from valuable liquids and sends the waste matter to the colon and the fluids to the kidney for further processing.

The Heart and Small Intestine have the following diagnostically significant Five Phase correspondences as they are assigned to the Fire Phase: the summer season, the climatic condition of heat, the color red, the emotion of happiness, the bitter taste, and the sound of laughter.

KIDNEY AND BLADDER

The Kidney in Chinese medicine is unquestionably a very special Organ. Tradition says that there is, as is the case for all other organs, only one kidney. The right kidney is called the Gate of Life, and is considered the storehouse of the original Prenatal Qi, which is the primary life force of the body. This *qi* enters into the process of circulation of *qi*, it is, in fact, the driving force of this circulation, and also enters into all the processes of the body that involve the creation or modification of energy. It is easy to lose, through drugs, excess sexuality, insufficient or excess sleep, improper diet, and poor living habits in general, and its loss is the ultimate reason for death. It is easy to dissipate but difficult to increase. It can, however, be increased by certain specific meditative techniques, as well as by the proper and repeated practice of Qi Kung, the Taoist equivalent of Hatha Yoga's pranayama, or energy control breathing exercises.

The Kidney controls the whole of the genitourinary area and is the basis for treatment of such diverse conditions as lumbago, prostatitis, uterine congestion, incontinence of urine, impotency, and inability to conceive. The uterus, one of the minor organs (along with the brain), is under the control of the Kidney. The Kidney enters into a special relationship with the heart, a fact not overlooked by our Western allopathic doctors. Its sense organ is the ear, and not only does the slow creeping of deafness in older people reflect the loss of Prenatal Qi and the weakening of the Kidneys, but, under non-degenerative conditions, deafness often can be treated effectively by using the Kidney as the basis of treatment.

The Kidney contains original essence acquired from the parent and acquired essence derived from the essence of food. Original essence defines the cycle of growth, maturity, and decay, and, of course, reproduction. Acquired essence (called Jing Qi) also forms marrow, which supplies the bones and the spinal column, and forms the brain. Although Jing Qi has general qualities as indicated, it has a specific manifestation as sperm.[9]

The qi sent to the Kidney by the Descending action of the Lung is then divided by the Yang of the Kidney into pure and impure fluids. Thus, the Kidney is in control of water metabolism. It also assists in the reception and spreading of qi through the body, and its condition is reflected in the hair of the head.

The major function of the urinary bladder is the temporary storage and excretion of the impure fluids in the form of urine. This is controlled by the Kidney.

The Kidney and Urinary Bladder have the following diagnostically significant Five Phase correspondences as they are assigned to the Water Phase: the winter season, the cold climatic condition, the color black, the emotion of fear, the salty taste, and the sound of groaning.

The Arm and Leg Lesser Yin channels of the Heart and Kidney surround the Great Yang channels of the Small Intestine and Urinary Bladder. They are the second set of four channels in the primary energy circulation. The energy is most prominent in the Heart from 11 A.M. to 1 P.M., in the Small Intestine from 1 to 3 P.M., in the Bladder from 3 to 5 P.M., and in the Kidney from 5 to 7 P.M.

HEART ENVELOPE AND SAN JIAO (THREE HEATERS)

These are function channels, which have no Western organ counterparts.[10] Although they are assigned to the element Fire, the Fire is of lesser consequence than the other pair of Fire Organs, and so they are considered to be Minister Fire to the Heart/Small Intestine Sovereign Fire. The distinction between the two lies in the relationship of the terms sovereign to minister; the minister is subordinate to and assists or serves the sovereign, which is primary. The San Jiao, commonly known as Three Heaters or Triple Warmer system, is said to be manifest as three areas or groupings of organs. The Lung and Heart are the upper warmer, the Stomach and Spleen are the middle warmer, and the Kidney and Colon are the lower warmer.

Sometimes the Small Intestine and the Liver are included as part of the lower warmer. The vascular system is probably the system over which the Heart Envelope Channel exercises control. These two are discussed at length in the section "Comments on the Names of the Pathways of Qi."

The Heart Envelope and San Jiao have the same correspondences as the Heart and Small Intestine.

LIVER AND GALL BLADDER   Strong negative emotions such as anger, rage, and deep depression are states which are both the result and the cause of difficulties in this organ pair. Anger and self-righteous behavior are met in America with the phrase "You've got a lot of gall." In Germany, short-tempered and self-righteous behavior is met with the phrase "A flea must have crawled over his liver." Both expressions, from two different continents, indicate the common awareness of the Liver/Gall Bladder relationship to these strong negative states. The Liver opens into the eyes, and Liver conditions are reflected in the eyes. The condition of exophthalmia (or "bug-eyes") is indicative of the rising of excess Fire in the Liver, and clearly an indication of strong emotional instability, in addition to its other clinical implications. Headaches also are often associated with Liver Fire in excess. Depression and frustration upset the spreading function of the Liver and lead to further depression, frustration, and bad temper.[11] The pulse of the Gall Bladder found on the left radial artery at the level of the styloid process of the wrist in the superficial position (felt with little or no pressure) will be pounding relative to the other pulses felt under the other fingers whenever a person either is in the process of manifesting negativity, or is repressing strong negative emotions.

The Liver stores blood and is responsible for nourishing and moistening. Failure of this moistening function is reflected in dry and painful eyes with blurred vision, difficulty in movement (including joint pain or stiffness), or dry skin. It stores and regulates the volume of circulating blood, holding part of the blood when the body is at rest. It cooperates with the heart in this blood-controlling function.

The Liver shares the responsibility for the distribution of qi with the Lung, thereby controlling certain vital functions including emotional changes, the functioning of the channels, and the organs, particularly the spleen and stomach, as well as bile secretion by the gall bladder. The Liver controls the sinews (muscles, joints, and particularly tendons), and its health is reflected in the nails. Finally, it controls the lower abdomen (the lower warmer), and is therefore important in the menstrual cycle.

The Gall Bladder stores and secretes gall, or bile. It is involved with the Heart in the decision-making process. It is interesting to contemplate the effect of this Yang Bowel's involvement in mental processes. Does it explain why human institutions are misused, abused, and corrupted? Is it the angry influence of the unhealthy Western Gall Bladder, due to the excess of fat ingestion in the Western world, that leads to the highly charged and far-reaching negative decisions that are so often made by our leaders?

The Liver and the Gall Bladder Channels show the following diagnostically significant Five Phase correspondences as they are assigned to the Wood Phase: the spring season, the climatic condition of wind, the color green, the angry emotion, the sour taste, and the sound of shouting.

The absolute Yin of the Arm and Leg, the Heat Envelope, and the Liver Channels surround the Lesser Yang Channels of the San Jiao and the Gall Bladder. These constitute the last set of four channels in the primary circulation of the energy. The energy is at "high tide" in the Heart Envelope from 7 to 9 P.M., in the San Jiao from 9 to 11 P.M., in the Gall Bladder from 11 P.M. to 1 A.M., and in the Liver from 1 to 3 A.M. The cycle begins again in the Lung at 3 A.M. Based upon traditional teachings about the speed of movement of *qi* through the channels, there are actually twenty-five circulations of the energy during the twenty-four hour period, but the "Organ Clock," as the Nutrient Cycle is often called, is concerned with the prominent tides of energy in each of the functional areas of the orbs. It should be noted that the time of weakest energy occurs from eleven to thirteen hours after the period of maximum activity.

The Creation of Energy, Pure Fluids, and Blood

Once again let us mention that the Prenatal Qi, which we shall call Kidney Essence, remains in the Kidney and is slowly depleted in the natural order of life. Its active part, Yuan Qi, begins to function at the moment of birth, when the lung begins to breathe, and the Lung, under the stimulus of Yuan Qi, starts the process of extraction of the Qi of Air from the inhaled substance.[12] Once food and drink enter the stomach, the process of separation of the Qi of Grain begins in the

Middle Warmer, and the Spleen transmits the Qi of Grain to the lung in the Upper Warmer, where it is combined with the Qi of Air, again under the influence of Yuan Qi, to form basic Nutrient Qi. Once this is activated by the Yuan Qi, the Nutrient Qi is formed and can move through the organ complex. This movement follows the traditional Five Phase pattern, traveling from the Lung to the Kidney and on to the Liver, the Heart and the Spleen, and back to the Lung. Each of the Viscera utilizes whatever is necessary for its own function, and passes part of the Nutrient Qi into the pertaining channel, where we shall call it Nourishing Qi, some into Defensive Qi, and the balance in the Five Phase circulation. Part of the Nutrient Qi is stored in the Kidney for emergency use.

Parallel to the process of energy transformation and transmission is the separation of pure fluids from the substance of food and drink that is passed by the stomach to the small intestine. The process begins in the small intestine, which then passes on the dregs to the colon, which attempts to salvage fluids for reprocessing. The fluids from the small intestine are passed to the kidney, where the pure and impure fluids are separated. The impure fluids are passed to the urinary bladder for excretion, while the pure fluid is processed and begins a circulation parallel to the circulation of *qi* through the organ complex. The circulation starts in the Kidney, where the pure fluid takes the form of parotid serous (serum), and continues to the Liver, where it is transformed into tears; into the Heart, which converts it to sweat; into the Spleen, where it produces saliva; and then into the Lung, where it becomes mucus. Under the control of the Defensive Qi, it is used to lubricate joints and sinews.

In addition to its other functions, the Spleen utilizes part of the Pure Fluid and part of the Nutritive Qi for the creation of Blood. The Blood is more energy than matter, except when its most Yin part takes the form of a literal fluid as it flows in the blood vessels. Much of the Blood flows in the channels with the Nourishing Qi, and is much more energetic than material.

Comments on the Names of the Pathways of Qi

Although most of the channels have names associated with their pertaining organs, and therefore the common abbreviations for the channels have tended to be abbreviations of the pertaining organ names, a few of the channels may have a number of different names connected to them. This has led to a certain confusion about which channel is the channel of reference and what the function of the channel may be as indicated by the name used. The nature of the channel energy and the significance of the energies are discussed elsewhere in the text, and an attempt to clarify names will be the primary purpose of this section, although in so doing we will introduce a number of important ideas about the Chinese view of the functions.

Each channel is named for its location on the arm or leg; its energetic quality (one of the six differentiations of the Yin/Yang polarity); and its pertaining organ or function (Lung, Heart, Liver, and others). In most cases this is a rather simple and straightforward task, with little or no variation possible in the names. In the two rather odd function-oriented channels, this problem has become complicated by assumptions about the information available to the ancient Chinese doctors, and the imposition of Western medical viewpoints on the Oriental medical model. We will first list the names, and, where existent, variations on the names of the organ-related channels and abbreviations of the channel names, and then attempt an explanation of the two function-related channels.

> The Arm Great Yin Lung Channel is abbreviated Lu (utilizing the first and second letters of the term Lung to establish the abbreviation)
>
> The Leg Great Yin Spleen Channel—Sp
>
> The Arm Lesser Yin Heart Channel—Ht
>
> The Leg Lesser Yin Kidney Channel—Ki
>
> The Arm Bright Yang Large Intestine Channel—Co (colon)—LI (Co is preferred for Large Intestine to avoid confusion with the "Li" of the liver).
>
> The Leg Bright Yang Stomach Channel—St
>
> The Arm Great Yang Small Intestine Channel—SI
>
> The Leg Great Yang Urinary Bladder Channel—UB—Bl
>
> The Leg Lesser Yang Gall Bladder Channel—GB
>
> The Leg Absolute Yin Liver Channel—Li—Lv—Liv
>
> The Arm Absolute Yin Heart Envelope Channel—HE
>
> The Arm Lesser Yang San Jiao—SJ

The Arm Absolute Yin Channel is the first of the two difficult-to-comprehend channels of *qi*. In Chinese, the name of the so-called pertaining organ is Hsin Pao Lo, which translates literally as The Envelope of the Heart. Early translators assumed that the Chinese medical practitioners were referring to the pericardium, the membrane which does indeed surround the heart. Western science is quite aware of the existence of the peritoneum, or the membrane which surrounds and holds the organs. A membrane surrounding a bone is called periosteum (around the bone), and the peritoneum of the heart is named specifically as the pericardium (around the heart). Thus the original name chosen for this channel was Pericardium Channel. With time and study it became clear that Chinese medical science was not concerned with, and probably not aware of, the existence of the pericardium, and if they were aware of these membranes, they were taken as part of the organ and given no individual significance. As time passed, it was observed repeatedly in clinical practice that the primary effect of treatment on this odd channel produced effects on the sexual function as well as on vascular circulation, and the channel was often called the Circulation-Sex Channel. With the increased recognition of the channel's effects on the circulatory system, there grew a recognition that that which enveloped the Heart was indeed the circulatory system, and that the sphere of influence of the channel extended deeply into the circulatory function, which accounted for the channel's effects on sexual function. Somehow, the term Heart Constrictor began to be used, as well as the more logical term Envelope of the Heart. Subsequently, Dr. R. Reinhold Voll showed that the points of the channel located on the hand were capable of very specific and direct influence of the major aspects of the vascular function, including the arteries, the veins, and others. The following list of abbreviated names are all used to describe this channel: P, HC, CX, EH, HE, and, most recently Cir. These refer, respectively, to Pericardium, Heart Constrictor, Circulation-Sex, Envelope of the Heart, Heart Envelope, and finally Circulation. EH or Cir would probably be best, but only time will tell which will become the standard.

The second channel which has caused difficulties is the Arm Lesser Yang Channel. In Chinese, the pertaining organ (or function) is called San Jiao, Three Burning Spaces, or Three Cauldrons, since there is a basis in Taoist philosophy for this name. In an effort to correlate this channel to Western anatomical functions, it was suggested that it related to the heat regulatory function of the Isles of Wills. This was a valiant attempt with little to recommend it in clinical evaluation, and it further

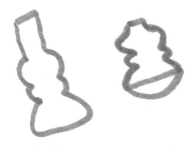

showed no real base in literature. The Three Burning Spaces were subsequently correlated to various Chinese medical concepts, as more and more literature became available. In Chinese medical thought, the body is divided into Upper, Middle, and Lower Heaters; Heater and Burning Space are used interchangeably. The Upper Burner consists of the Lungs and Heart, the Middle Burner of the Stomach and Spleen, and the Lower Burner of the Kidney and Colon. Bladder, Liver, and Small Intestine are also considered part of the Lower Burner. This grouping demonstrates the functional role of the Arm Absolute Yin Channel as the controller of the three processes of Digestion, Assimilation, and Elimination. It must, of course, be recognized that Chinese medicine regards the Spleen as primarily the controller of the Digestive Function. Thus, digestion takes place in the Stomach, where tradition says that the Qi of Grain is separated from the substance of food, under the control of the Spleen. From here the Qi of Grain passes into the Lung, where it mingles with the Qi of Air to become the Nutrient Qi of the body. Under the control of the Heart, it is then distributed throughout the organism. Thus, the Upper Warmer controls Assimilation. Finally, the impure solids pass into the Colon, and the impure fluids into the Kidney and Bladder for Elimination. There is no question about the clinical use of the channel for this very valid purpose in treating conditions of the human organism.

Recognizing the Taoist spiritual influence in the channel name Three Cauldrons, or Burning Spaces, a number of acupuncturists began to explore the channel to affect the *shen* (or spirit) and found great clinical value in the treatment of emotional distress and emotional accompaniments to disease conditions through this channel. The research of Dr. Reinhold Voll and his colleagues in Germany shows the effect of certain hand points of the Arm Lesser Yang Channel. Points were discovered which had powerful and direct influence on specific Endocrine Glands. Dr. Voll's work enabled acupuncturists and advanced Amma therapists to treat dysfunctions related to the Endocrine Glands with a new level of accomplishment.

Thus, the orb is seen to influence three major areas: the processes of Digestion, Assimilation, and Elimination; Emotional Factors; and the functions of Endocrine Glands, leading to the following abbreviated names for the channel: TH, TW, SJ, End, which are, respectively, Three Heaters, Triple Warmer, San Jiao, and Endocrine Channel. SJ is slowly becoming the preferred usage in the American acupuncture community.

The Pathways of Qi for the Amma Therapist

Most books and charts which intend to teach the concepts of Oriental manipulative therapy show the superficial branches of the principal pathways of *qi*. These do indeed have great significance for the acupuncturist, who uses the loci (points) on the superficial branches of the main channels to assist in diagnosis and as the primary points of treatment, as well as to the advanced Amma therapist, who uses them primarily for evaluative purposes. Rarely discussed are the internal pathways of the channels and the particular type of channels which are generally used for treatment by the Amma therapist. This has resulted in a serious misunderstanding of the true nature of the art of Oriental manipulative therapy. We do not wish the same fate to occur to the mother of all commonly known Oriental manipulative techniques, the science of Amma therapy.

PROPER NOMENCLATURE FOR THE PATHWAYS OF QI

For a long time there was a paucity of English translations of Chinese medical literature available to the acupuncturist and to the would-be therapist, and a complete absence of literature on traditional Oriental manipulative therapy, save a few very basic books outlining the art of Shiatsu from Japan. The result was the mistaken idea that the twelve bilateral meridians ("imaginary lines"), and the two midline vessels ("closed containers") constituted the defined scope of the system, and were used by acupuncturists and manipulative therapists alike. Also the misnomer acupressure ("acu"-needle) come into use based on the assumption that the therapist treated the same "imaginary lines" as the acupuncturist. A far more conceptually correct term for the pathways of *qi* is "channel" rather than meridians or vessels. They are the pathways through which energy flows throughout the body. In fact, the pathways of *qi* are neither imaginary lines on the surface of the body, nor closed vessels containing some fluid energy. The term "channel" implies a pathway which can increase and decrease, ebb and flow, stagnate and rush, or diminish and overflow. This is, indeed, a more proper understanding of the bioenergetic system, which is the basis of Amma therapy and related Oriental medical arts.

QI AS AN EXPERIMENTALLY VERIFIABLE PHYSICAL EVENT

The bioenergy enlivens the physical form. According to the Bharta Dharma (the philosophy of India), to interact with the world, the mind uses a dual system made of the Manomaya Kosha (the body of food) and the Pranamaya Kosha (the body of energy), and these two taken together are called the living physical body. The channels of *qi* constitute that bioenergy or Pranamaya Kosha, which is without doubt a complex and active system. It has been described in great detail in Chinese literature, with the same kind of scientific study and precision as any Western anatomy, insofar as was possible with primitive measuring instruments of ancient China.

Today, sponsored by the new government of China, extensive research into the nature of the channels is being actively pursued, and numerous corroborations of traditional views have resulted from such studies. Studies at the University of Toronto, the New Center for Wholistic Health Education and Research, UCLA, and other American institutions, and numerous studies abroad, have begun to clearly corroborate the Chinese view of the polar bioenergy. Modern allopathic physicians can have no quarrel with the basic concept of bioenergy, as they recognize the bioelectrical activity of the nervous system, the signals in the heart and elsewhere, and the greater and lesser areas of bioelectrical potential both on the surface and within the body. The major difference between the results of Western and Eastern research lies in the application of observation and theory to the bioenergy to discover and understand the nature of the patterns of the flow of *qi* and its relation to disease and health. However, Western medicine has still to explore bioenergy in relation to the flow of *qi* and its influence on health and disease. Only in the last fifty years has any serious study been undertaken in the West on the nature and significance of bioenergy. Of course, the works of Wilhelm Reich, Baron Von Richenbacker, and the magnetic healers, which were often ridiculed by the simplistic and narrow scientific establishment of the times, should not be overlooked for the depth of their understanding and their effort in the face of a hostile environment.[13]

PROPER NAMES FOR THE CHANNELS

As a result of the original and limited translations of the Chinese texts, it has become common practice to name the channels by their major pertaining organ. This is a very poor choice of terms, as it has led to a misunderstanding of the whole channel system. As discussed in the section on Yin/Yang, the Chinese, in fact, name the channels in relation to the six energies which are the six transitory phases of the manifestation of Yin/Yang.

The six energies are symbolized in Figure 1; which also shows which of the channels carries each differentiation of the energy, the basic quality of the channel as indicated by its element, the channel's pertaining organ, and whether it flows superficially on the upper or lower limb. A brief digression here on the pattern of flow would not be out of order. The flow of qi is obviously continuous in the body, but it shows clear patterns of ebb and flow, and of increase and decrease, and these patterns correlate to western observations of functional physiology.

The Path of qi, the basic pattern of flow through the main channels and therefore the basic pattern of qi flow in the organism, begins at 3 A.M., when the Great Yin begins to rise, and peaks at 4 A.M., when its qi drops off rapidly, passing into its opposite, the Bright Yang. As the qi flows down from the upper torso, it peaks in the Arm Bright Yang Large Intestine Channel at 6 A.M. and then again in the Leg Bright Yang Stomach Channel at 8 A.M., where it returns to the Great Yin of the Leg, whose pertaining organ is the Spleen. Part of the qi continues to circulate back into the Arm Great Yin Lung Channel, continuing the pattern of the duality of the Bright Yang and Great Yin. A tertiary flow continues between the Arm and Leg couples, the Bright Yang Large Intestine and the Great Yin Lung Channels, as well as between the Great Yin Spleen and the Bright Yang Stomach Channels. Much of the basis for treatment lies in the relationships established in the secondary and tertiary pathways. The primary pathway of qi, also called the Nutrient Cycle, continues through the next group of four in a similar manner, and finally through the third group of four. This constitutes a full twenty-four-hour cycle of the tides in the Path of qi. There are twenty-five full cycles of the energy in twenty-four hours, but the tides are as indicated. The process is summarized in table 2.

	Channel	Pertaining Organ	Period of Maximum Activity
TABLE 2	Arm Great Yin	Lung	3 A.M. ‹ 4 A.M.› 5 A.M.
	Arm Bright Yang	Large Intestine	5 A.M. ‹ 6 A.M.› 7 A.M.
	Leg Bright Yang	Stomach	7 A.M. ‹ 8 A.M.› 9 A.M.
	Leg Great Yin	Spleen	9 A.M. ‹10 A.M.› 11 A.M.
	Arm Lesser Yin	Heart	11 A.M. ‹12 P.M.› 1 P.M.
	Arm Great Yang	Small Intestine	1 P.M. ‹ 2 P.M.› 3 P.M.
	Leg Great Yang	Urinary Bladder	3 P.M. ‹ 4 P.M.› 5 P.M.
	Leg Lesser Yin	Kidney	5 P.M. ‹ 6 P.M.› 7 P.M.
	Arm Absolute Yin	Heart Envelope	7 P.M. ‹ 8 P.M.› 9 P.M.
	Arm Lesser Yang	Three Warmers	9 P.M. ‹10 P.M.› 11 P.M.
	Leg Lesser Yang	Gall Bladder	11 P.M. ‹12 A.M.› 1 A.M.
	Leg Absolute Yin	Liver	1 A.M. ‹ 2 A.M.› 3 A.M.

THE ANATOMY OF THE PATHWAYS OF QI

In brief, the system called Ching-Lou, the channels and collaterals, consists of the complex of energy pathways that enliven every area of the body. First, the twelve major internal pathways wind and unite through the total organism, pass through the major organs, and branch into the superficial regions of the body. These superficial branches are the channels upon which the acupuncturist locates his points and inserts needles to a depth of between one-eighth and four inches to make contact with the *qi* of the main channels. Second, lying within the deeper regions of the body, and extending the range of effect of the main channels, are the Twelve Divergent Channels. Arising at the connecting points of the main channels are the Transverse Lou or Connecting Channels, which are short branches between coupled main channels, as well as the Longitudinal Lou Channels, which act as reservoirs of channel *qi* and further extend the distribution of *qi*. Connecting and regulating the Yin and Yang channels separately, and binding all the channels at the transverse midline of the body, are the Eight Extraordinary Channels. Enlivening and feeding the muscles and tendons are the Tendino-Muscle Channels, which form a more superficial network at the level of the muscles, with some deeper branches connecting internally to the spine, the ribs, and the tongue. And finally, we have arrived at the surface, at the Twelve Cutaneous Regions, the superficial residence of the *qi* of the channels. This brief explanation is given to show the complexity of the system.

Most of the channels and their branches disperse into broad webs of energy, not unlike the capillaries of the vascular system. Like the neurological and vascular systems, the bioenergy system, when isolated from the rest of the body, shows the shape and size of the whole. And just as the neurological and vascular systems disperse disease deeper and deeper into the body as well as carry internal and external healing substances the channels of *qi* act to defend, protect, and nourish the whole while still allowing perverse energy access to the deeper regions of the body.

Figures 3 through 14 show the superficial and deep pathways of the Primary Organ Channels. The superficial pathways are of great value for reference in studying the Tendino-Muscle Channels, since the former flow through the latter. Note also the direction of the flow of *qi*. Yang Qi flows down from Heaven (in the Chinese anatomical position, the arms are always raised), and Yin flows up from the Earth. Sometimes this seems contradictory to superficial observation; it has even led to confusion among the advocates of the sometimes very useful macrobiotics. Yin is heavy and internal; Yang is light and external. Yin is the interior; Yang is the surface. These qualities of Yin and Yang often confuse the understanding of energy and its movements and qualities. If one keeps in mind the poetic concept that Yin is Earth and Yang is Heaven, and further, the concept of the transmutation of *qi* into its polar quality as indicated in the basic symbol of Yin/Yang, it will become apparent that Yang flows down from its source in Heaven, and in that downward flow is converted into its polar quality to take on various Yin forms on Earth. The Yin of the Earth flows up toward Heaven, and, undergoing like transformation, feeds the Qi of Heaven and nourishes the Yang.

Figures 15 and 16 show the two Midline Channels, the Governing Vessel Channel, and the Conception Vessel Channels, which are the only two of the Eight Extraordinary Channels to be mentioned in the text. These channels are significant in that they have branches to many other channels, to the Yin for the Conception Channel and to the Yang for the Governing Vessel Channel, as well as to the newly identified channels of German Electroacupuncture (electroacupuncture according to Voll). The Conception Channel controls the genitourinary area; this channel *qi* must be flowing for there to be conception. Control points for the functions of the Three Warmers are also found on this channel. The Governing Vessel Channel includes control points for each of the viscera, bowels, and several other functions.

Figures 17 to 28 are rather detailed illustrations of the Tendino-Muscle Channels, including several branches not generally indicated in the academic literature, and some modifications in the traditional academic view of the exact pathways. These corrections are the result of nearly forty years of training, study, and almost constant practice by Mrs. Sohn, whose qualifications have been described elsewhere in this book. It is quite possible that the pathways are somewhat modified as a result of time, or it may reflect differences in the population of patients. The ancient texts are based on the study and treatment of the ancient Chinese, and Mrs. Sohn's work is based on the study and treatment of modern Koreans and Americans. Please remember that all references in this text relative to pathways, treatments, and pressures are relative to the Tendino-Muscle Channels, and are not to be confused with the much narrower and far less accessible superficial branches of the main channels. Some modern books on Oriental medical arts have presented the thesis that the Tendino-Muscle Channels are a reference to the network of tendons and muscles that coat the underlying viscera, nerves, and bones. Although the Nutrient Qi of the muscular system as well as the Defensive Qi on the surface is delivered by the Tendino-Muscle Channels, it is not accurate to identify the channel system with the physical form of the muscles. More than one Tendino-Muscle Channel is often found to feed the same muscle, and the channels are found to be far thinner than the muscles through which they move, such as the branches of the Bladder Tendino-Muscle Channel over the gluteal region. They are, however, the major channels of Defensive Qi and are responsible for the protection of the body energetically, as are the muscles structurally.

Figures 29 to 31 show the Six (or as some would prefer, the Twelve) Cutaneous Regions, the areas on the surface, from the superficial aspect of the Tendino-Muscle Channels through to the very superficial aspects of the dermis, which reflect the six basic differentiations of the primary Yin/Yang polarities. They are called Twelve Cutaneous Regions to correspond to the Arm and Leg aspects of the six forms of energy.

This explanation should be sufficient for the beginning therapist to initiate an exploration of the nature of the channel system, and to comprehend how stimulation of the superficial aspects of the body may have profound effects deep within the organism.

POINTS USED IN
APPLICATION OF PRESSURE
IN AMMA

Acupuncture points found on the superficial branches are not the basis of Amma therapy; however, a certain class of points is shared by the acupuncturist and the Amma therapist, and these points are traditionally known as Ah Shui points, which translates roughly as "ouch!" For the treatment of such conditions as sciatica, tendinitis, muscular pulls, and strains, the acupuncturist palpates for tender spots on the Tendino-Muscle Channels and needles these points (if they are not directly over an artery or nerve) with amazing and rapid results. This is the real method of point choice for the primary and midlevel Amma therapist. Thus, the so-called acupressure, the stimulation of acupuncture points with the fingers, is not an accurate description of this method of treatment, and pressure on acupuncture points is a method of stimulation used by acupuncturists only if needles, moxa, or even electrotherapy is not available. Proper pressure applied to Ah Shui points is the preferred method of treatment. It may be noted here that the study of trigger point therapy, which was originally applied to musculo-skeletal problems, in some cases parallels both superficial channel points and Ah Shui points. Trigger point therapy is not, however, parallel to Amma therapy conceptually, nor are the majority of the points used contiguous with those used by the Amma therapist. It is not surprising that many loci on the body will be within the limits of practical application of a number of different systems.

A SUMMARY OF THE FLOW PATTERNS OF THE QI

As the Pathways of Qi are complex and rather numerous, it should be helpful to summarize here the most important flow patterns.

Qi Cycles in the Channels:

The Nutrient Cycle	Begins in the Lung and flows as follows: Lu Co St Sp Ht SI Bl KI HE SJ GB Liv.
The Yin/Yang Pairs	Each coupled set of inner/outer channels has an independent flow through the mediation of the lateral *lou* channels. Each pair is of the same Five-Phase quality: Lu/Co; St/Sp; Ht/SI; Bl/KI; HE/SJ; GB/Liv.
The Arm/Leg Pairs	Because the channels are paired in the flow of each of the Six Chiao, there are strong influences between the arm and leg branches of each of the six energy types: Lu/Sp; Co/St; Ht/Ki; SI/Bl; HE/Liv; SJ/GB.
The Tendino-Muscle Channels	It is often said by acupuncturists that these channels carry only Defensive Qi. If this were so, there would be no method for distribution of Nutrient Qi to the superficial regions. It is probable that the Defensive Qi flows primarily in these channels for twenty-five cycles during the day and in closer proximity with the inner pathways at night for twenty-five cycles.
The Midline Channels	Although little mention has been made of this rather significant pair of the Eight Extraordinary Channels, it is necessary to mention that they have many connections to other channels, the Governing Vessel Channel to the Yang and the Conception Vessel Channel to the Yin, and that there is a distinct circulation between the two, which is the subject of much study in esoteric and modern scientific circles.

Qi cycles in the Viscera:

The Creation Cycle	follows the outer Five Element pattern: Ht Sp Lu Ki Liv.
The Control Cycle	follows the inner Five Element pattern: Ht Lu Liv Sp Ki.

The Primary Organ Channels

ARM GREAT YIN *LUNG*
METAL CHANNEL

DEEP—This channel begins in the Middle Burner, deep to CV 12. It descends to loop around the transverse colon. It then ascends, passing the cardiac orifice of the stomach, where the stomach and the esophagus meet. The channel pierces the diaphragm, then enters into the lungs. It moves up toward the throat and then crosses the upper thorax

SUPERFICIAL—The channel surfaces approximately one *tsun* (acupuncture unit of measurement) below the lateral aspect of the clavicle, in the second intercostal space, lateral to the mammillary line. It then descends the upper arm, following a pathway that falls between the long and short heads of the biceps brachii. Lu 5 lies lateral to the biceps tendon at the elbow fold. The channel continues in its descent, passing between the brachioradialis and the pronator teres to the anterior margin of the styloid process of the radius. It crosses the wrist fold, continuing between the opponens pollicis and the abductor pollicis brevis to the radial side of the nail root of the thumb, where this channel ends at Lu 11.

A DEEP branch splits from Lu 7, just proximal to the wristfold above the styloid process, and crosses over the dorsum of the hand to the radial aspect of the nail bed of the index finger to communicate with Co 1.

Figure 3   Arm Great Yin *Lung* Metal Channel

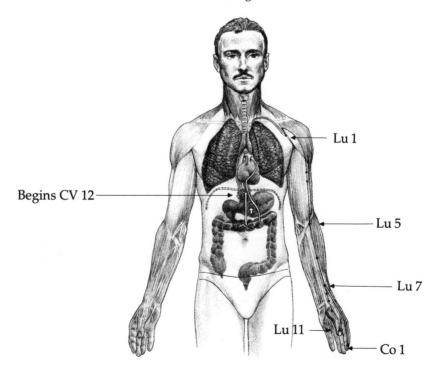

Arm Bright Yang *Colon* Metal Channel

Figure 4

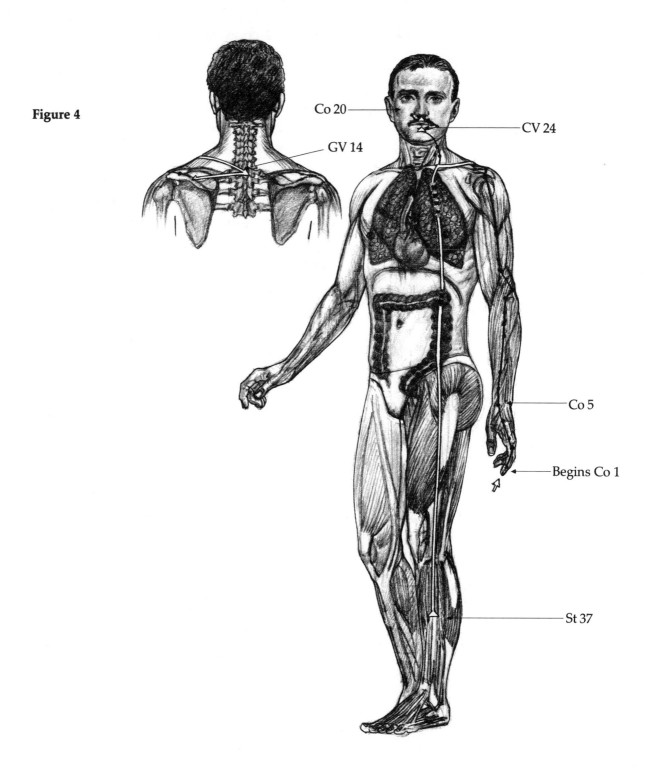

Co 20

CV 24

GV 14

Co 5

Begins Co 1

St 37

ARM BRIGHT YANG *COLON* METAL CHANNEL

SUPERFICIAL—The Colon Channel begins on the radial edge of the index finger. It passes through the first and second metacarpal bones, moving through the depression between the tendons of the extensor pollicis longus (on the ulnar side of the dorsal surface of the hand) and the extensor pollicis brevis and abductor pollicis (on the radial border of the dorsum of the hand). This is known as the "anatomical snuffbox," and it is here that Co 5 is found. The channel ascends along the posterolateral border of the extensor digitorum, over the supinator longus, and toward the elbow fold. Co 11 is located on the lateral epicondyle of the humerus. It follows the lateral aspect of the triceps to the acromio-clavicular articulation. Between the acromion and the head of the humerus lies Co 15.

DEEP—From here the channel moves medially and posteriorly across the anterior aspect of the acromion to GV (Governing Vessel) 14, between C7 and T1. It moves anteriorly and enters the supraclavicular fossa, where St 12 is found. The channel splits here, a deep pathway descending into the thoracic cavity, and a superficial pathway ascending into the neck and face. The DEEP branch descends, passing through the lung and the diaphragm, to the flexure of the colon (each bilateral branch of the Co channel descends to the associated flexure, i.e., the branch on the right passes to the hepatic flexure, and the branch on the left passes to the splenic flexure). A branch continues in its descent to St 37. From the supraclavicular fossa a SUPERFICIAL branch moves upward through the neck, crosses the cheek, and moves DEEP, entering into the lower gum. It curves around the lip and (SUPERFICIAL) intersects the same channel, coming from the opposite side, at the philtrum. The Co Channel ends at the ala of the nose at Co 20, where it connects with the Stomach Channel.

Leg Bright Yang *Stomach* Earth Channel

Figure 5

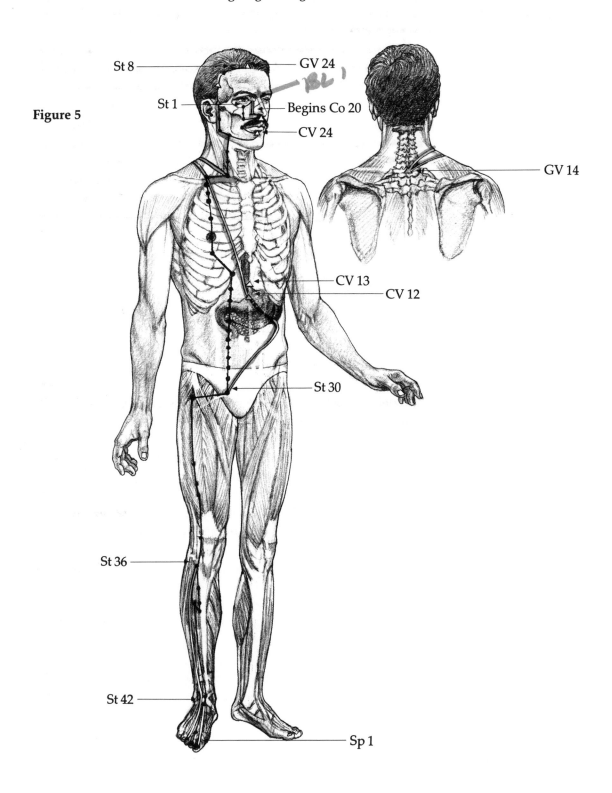

LEG BRIGHT YANG
STOMACH
EARTH CHANNEL

DEEP—This channel starts at Co 20 at the ala of the nose. It ascends the side of the nose to Bl 1 and then passes laterally to emerge SUPERFICIALLY at St 1, which lies vertically below the center of the pupil on the infraorbital margin, at which point a tiny sulcus can be palpated. It moves through St 2 and St 3, and moves DEEP to meet with GV at the labial frenum. It passes around the mouth to meet with CV 24 and then emerges SUPERFICIALLY at St 5 in the inferior border of the mandible in the facial artery groove. It passes laterally along the distal border of the jaw. The channel splits here, one branch ascending from the angle of the jaw, and one branch descending into the torso. The ascending branch passes along the angle of the jaw to St 8, which is found at the horizontal level of the superior hairline close to the coronal suture. It then moves DEEP to connect with GV 24.

SUPERFICIAL—The descending branch moves into the supraclavicular fossa. From here it moves DEEP to GV 14 and then emerges once again at (SUPERFICIAL) the supraclavicular fossa. Here it splits once again and descends into the torso in both a SUPERFICIAL and a DEEP branch. The SUPERFICIAL branch descends along the mammillary line, following the lateral margin of the rectus abdominus muscles, passing beside the umbilicus and through the lower abdomen to the inguinal region. The DEEP pathway runs internally parallel to the superficial channel. It pierces through the diaphragm, intersects with CV 13 and CV 12, and then drops into the stomach, spleen, and large intestine. The DEEP and SUPERFICIAL channels join at St 30, at the lateral margin of the pubis. (SUPERFICIAL) The channel leaves the torso at the horizontal level of the pubic bone, curving laterally toward the anterior aspect of the thigh where St 31 is found, lying in the apex of the angle formed by the sartorius and the tensor fascia latae. The channel continues in its descent following the interstice between the vastus lateralis and rectus femoris. It descends to ST 36 where it again splits. From St 36 a DEEP branch descends, terminating at the lateral edge of the third toe. From St 36 a SUPERFICIAL branch passes down along the lateral border of the tibia, passing over the dorsum of the foot between the second and third metatarsals, and ends at the lateral side of the distal phalange of the second toe. A branch separates from St 42 and terminates on the medial edge of the great toe where it connects with the Spleen Channel at Sp 1.

Leg Great Yin *Spleen* Earth Channel

Figure 6

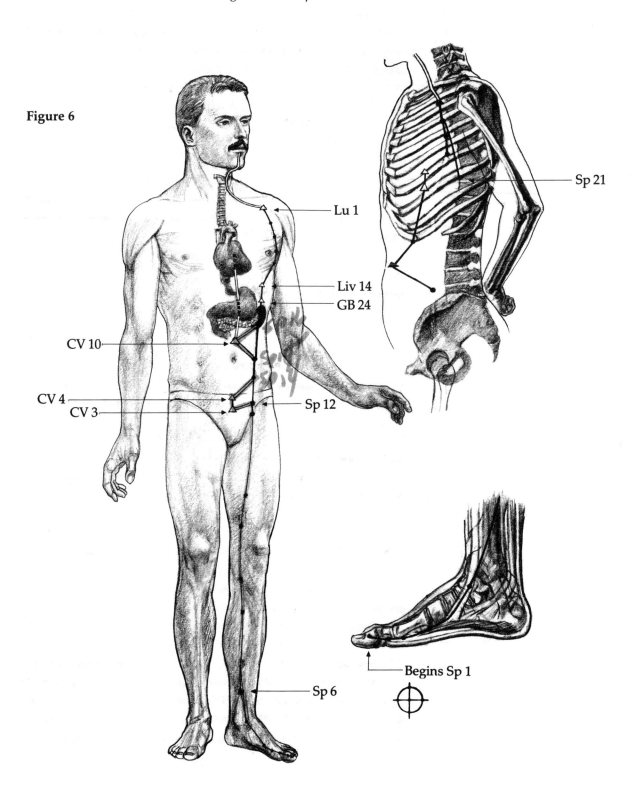

Lu 1

Liv 14

GB 24

CV 10

CV 4

CV 3

Sp 12

Sp 21

Begins Sp 1

Sp 6

LEG GREAT YIN *SPLEEN* EARTH CHANNEL

SUPERFICIAL—This pathway originates on the medial border of the most distal phalange of the great toe and moves along the most medial aspect of the foot at the meeting of the dorsal and plantar skins. It passes anterior to the medial malleolus, medial to the tendon of the tibialis anterior. The channel continues in its ascent up the leg, running along the posterior aspect of the tibia to the patella, and ascends the antero-medial thigh, travelling anterior to the Liver Channel. At the point where the channel reaches the inguinal fold, it is on the mammillary line, vertically below the nipple. Here the channel enters into the abdominal cavity. The pathway continues DEEP, intersecting CV 3 and CV 4. It surfaces to Sp 14 and Sp 15 SUPERFICIAL, and then moves DEEP once again, first to communicate with CV 10, and then to enter into its pertaining organ, the spleen, and to communicate with the stomach. It continues in its DEEP pathway passing through the diaphragm and dispersing into the heart. From the stomach region, the CV 10 area, a SUPERFICIAL branch passes through Sp 16 and intersects with Gall Bladder at GB 24 and Liver at Li 14. From here the channel continues to Sp 17–21. (Sp 21 is the endpoint of the SUPERFICIAL pathway. It is called the Universal Lou, the Great Regulator. From this point a capillary network ramifies over the whole body and commands energy in both Yin and Yang channels.) A branch moves from Sp 20 to intersect with Lu 1, and then to move DEEP to ascend along the esophagus, and to disperse into the root of the tongue and the lower lingual area.

Arm Lesser Yin *Heart* Fire Channel

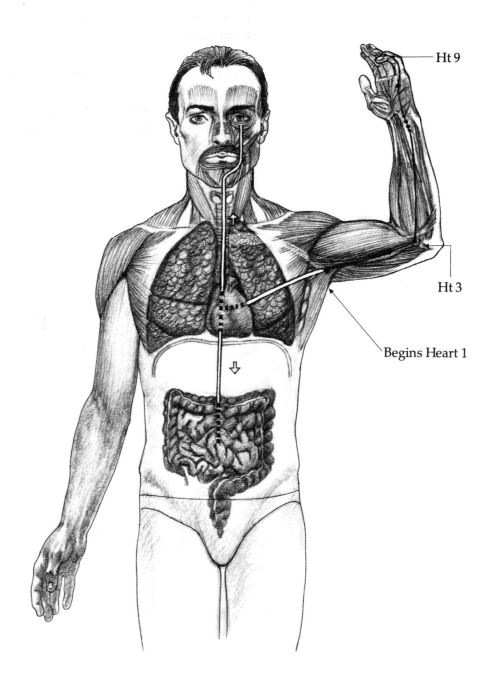

Figure 7

Ht 9

Ht 3

Begins Heart 1

ARM LESSER YIN *HEART* FIRE CHANNEL

DEEP—The Heart Channel begins in the heart. Here it divides into three branches. The descending branch passes through the diaphragm and connects to the small intestines. The ascending branch runs upward along the esophagus to the face, where it joins the tissues surrounding the eye. A third branch travels transversely from the heart to the lung and then emerges SUPERFICIALLY at the axilla. From here it passes along the posterior border of the medial aspect of the upper arm and descends in the interstice between the biceps brachii and the medial head of the triceps. It moves through the cubital fossa and between the pronator teres and the palmaris longus, and continues along the medial aspect of the forearm in the space between the palmaris longus and the flexor carpi ulnaris to the capitate bone proximal to the palm. The channel passes on the inside border of the hypothenar eminence, where it passes along the radial border of the fifth metacarpal. It ends at point Ht 9 at the radial edge of the nail root of the fifth digit.

Arm Great Yang *Small Intestine* Fire Channel

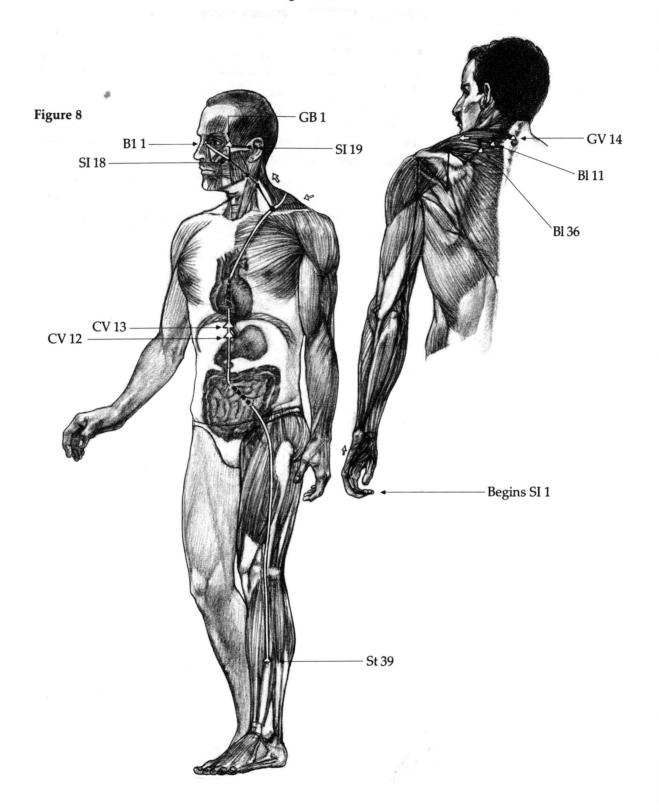

Figure 8

ARM GREAT YANG
SMALL INTESTINE
FIRE CHANNEL

SUPERFICIAL—This channel begins at the ulnar tip of the little finger. It ascends along the ulnar side of the dorsum of the hand to the wrist, where it passes the styloid process of the ulna. It ascends the postero-medial forearm, and passes between the olecranon of the ulna and the medial epicondyle of the humerus at the medial elbow. It proceeds along the posterior aspect of the upper arm, following the medial head of the triceps. It passes the superior aspect of the axillary fold of the upper arm and proceeds to the shoulder joint. The path turns toward the center of the infraspinatus fossa at the horizontal level of the fifth spinous process, where it then turns upward, moving above the superior border of the spine of the scapula. It continues medially, passing over the supraspinatus fossa and the medial border of the scapula, ascending toward the neck. At the top of the shoulder it crosses the Bladder Channel at Bl 36 and Bl 11. DEEP—It intersects with GV 14 at the level of the seventh cervical vertebra. It moves anteriorly into the supraclavicular fossa, where it divides into two branches. The DEEP branch descends into the torso to communicate with the heart. It continues in its descent along the esophagus, passing through the diaphragm to enter into the stomach and the channel's pertaining organ, the small intestine. In its descent the channel connects with the Conception Vessel at CV 12 and CV 13. This branch continues in its descent to intersect the Stomach Channel at ST 39. The SUPERFICIAL branch from the supraclavicular fossa ascends the neck and the cheek, moving to the outer canthus of the eye, where it meets the Gall Bladder Channel at GB 1. It turns posteriorly, crosses the temple, and enters the ear at SI 19. A branch separates from SI 18 on the cheek and ascends to the infraorbital region of the eye, where it meets Bl 1 at the inner canthus of the eye.

Leg Great Yang *Urinary Bladder* Water Channel

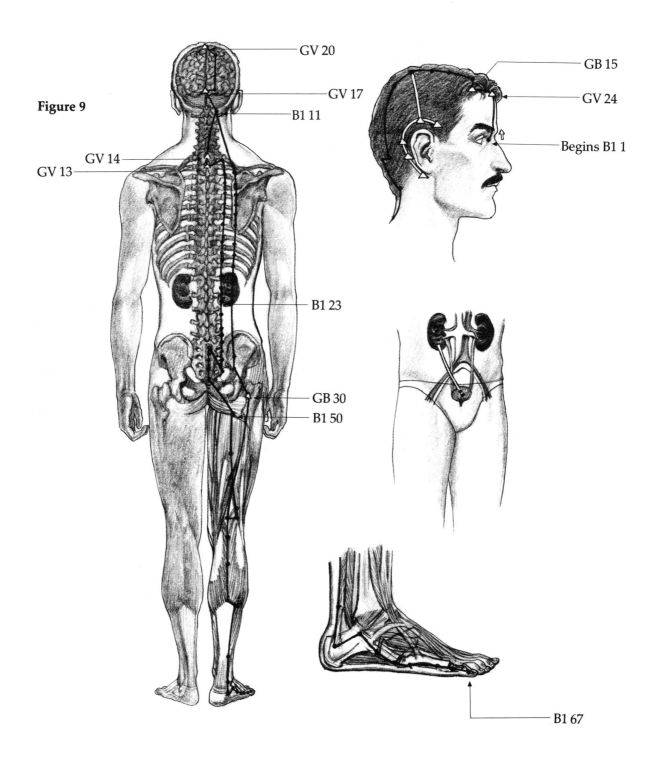

Figure 9

GV 20

GV 17

B1 11

GV 14

GV 13

B1 23

GB 30

B1 50

GB 15

GV 24

Begins B1 1

B1 67

LEG GREAT YANG
URINARY BLADDER
WATER CHANNEL

SUPERFICIAL—This channel begins at the inner canthus of the eye at Bl 1. It ascends the forehead, intersecting with the Governing Vessel Channel at GV 24 and with the Gall Bladder Channel at GB 15. It then crosses to the vertex and again intersects Governing Vessel at GV 20. From here a branch passes laterally to the area above the ear, joining Gall Bladder at GB 7, 8, and 12. From GV 20, another branch descends vertically into the brain and then joins with Governing Vessel at GV 17. The channel descends to Bl 10, where it bifurcates to descend along the nape of the neck in two parallel branches. From Bl 10 the medial branch descends to meet with the Governing Vessel at GV 14 and 13. It then moves upward to Bl 11 before descending, parallel to the spine, to the lumber region. DEEP—The channel enters into the internal cavity via the paravertebral muscles at the area of Bl 23, to communicate with the kidneys and finally with its associated organ, the bladder.

SUPERFICIAL—From the lumbar region, the branch crosses the buttock and descends to the popliteal fossa at the posterior aspect of the knee. From Bl 10 the second, lateral branch descends parallel to the spine along the medial border of the scapula to the gluteal region. It crosses the buttock, intersects with GB 30, and then descends along the lateral, posterior portion of the thigh to meet with the medial branch at the popliteal fossa. Together they run down the gastrocnemius muscle to the area behind the lateral malleolus. It then follows the fifth metatarsal to the lateral nail root of the fifth digit, where it ends at Bl 67. Here it will unite with the Kidney Channel.

Leg Lesser Yin *Kidney* Water Channel

Figure 10

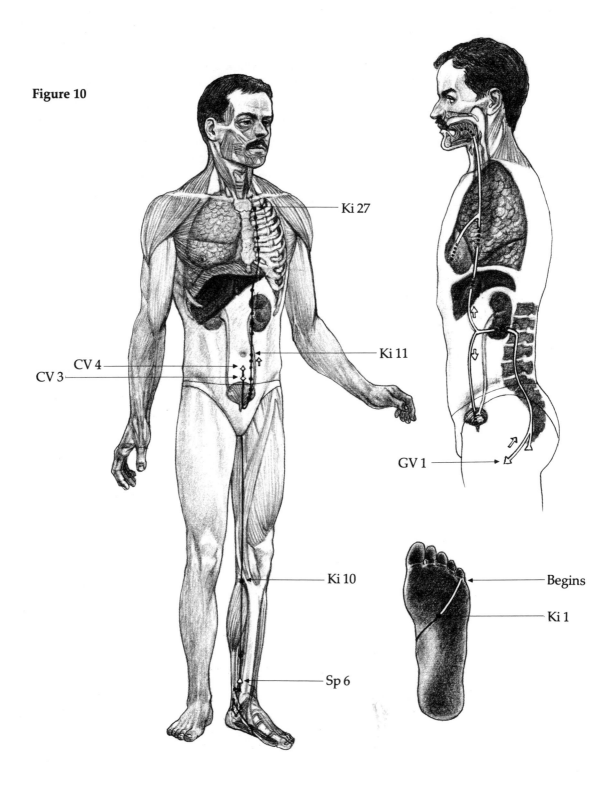

Ki 27

Ki 11

CV 4

CV 3

GV 1

Ki 10

Sp 6

Begins

Ki 1

LEG LESSER YIN *KIDNEY WATER CHANNEL*

PATHWAY—The Kidney Channel starts on the medial aspect of the fifth digit. It moves across the sole of the foot, passing to SUPERFICIAL Ki 1 at the border of the anterior third of the sole of the foot, between the second and third metatarso-phalangeal joints where the toes are flexed. From here it travels posterior to the medial malleolus, enters the heel, and proceeds upward along the medial aspect of the lower leg, where it unites with the Spleen and Liver Channels at Sp 6. It ascends the medial aspect of the leg within the gastrocnemius muscle to the medial aspect of the popliteal fossa. Ki 10 can be found between the tendons of the semitendinosus and the semimembranosus at the popliteal fossa. It continues to ascend the postero-medial aspect of the thigh to the base of the spine, DEEP, where it intersects GV 1 between the anus and the tip of the coccyx. Here it threads its way beneath the lumbar region of the spine, where it enters its associated organ, the kidney. Here the channel divides into two pathways. An ascending branch passes through the liver and the diaphragm, enters the lung, and then follows the throat to terminate at the root of the tongue. A branch separates from the lung, connects with the heart, and disperses into the chest, where it connects with Heart Envelope Channel. A descending branch from the kidney descends into the bladder. From the bladder organ the channel moves SUPERFICIALLY, to connect first with CV 4 and then CV 3, and then it emerges at Ki 11 to unite with *Chung Mei (Vital Vessel, or Penetrating Vessel)*. The *Chung Mei* or Penetrating Vessel plays a fundamental role in the deep circulation. It is known as the "Sea of Blood" because of the governing effect it has on menstruation. This explans the use of Kidney points for their influential effect on menses. The combined vessels then travel to Ki 21. The primary branch of the Kidney Channel continues from Ki 21, ascending over the most medial aspects of the intercostal spaces of the sixth, fifth, fourth, third, and second ribs to terminate at Ki 27, between the first and second ribs.

Arm Absolute Yin *Heart Envelope* Fire Channel

Figure 11

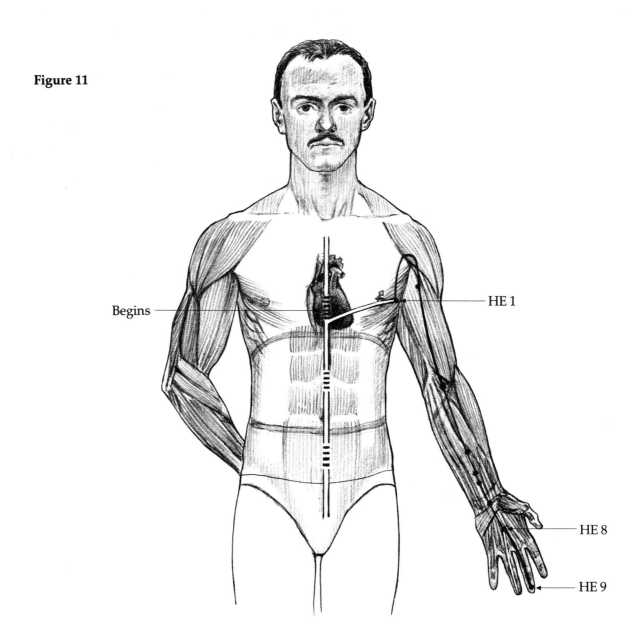

Begins

HE 1

HE 8

HE 9

ARM ABSOLUTE YIN
HEART ENVELOPE
FIRE CHANNEL

DEEP—This channel begins in the chest. It descends across the diaphragm and into the abdomen, where it connects successively with the upper, middle, and lower burners of the Triple Heater (San Jiao). A branch from the chest runs transversely to the costal region, where it emerges (SUPERFICIAL) at HE 1, located three *tsun* below the axillary fold, approximately one tsun lateral to the mammillary line in the fourth intercostal space. The channel then ascends to the axilla, where it descends along the medial aspect of the upper arm and between the two heads of the biceps branchii to the cubital fossa. From here it continues down the forearm between the tendons of the palmaris longus and the flexor carpi radialis. Entering the palm, it follows the middle finger to the radial nail root of the middle finger, where it ends at HE 9. Some texts give the location of HE 9 at the tip of the middle finger rather than at the radial nail root, but this is an irrelevant distinction for the Amma therapist. A DEEP branch separates in the palm from HE 8 and runs along the ring finger to the ulnar nail root, where it connects with San Jiao.

Arm Lesser Yang *San Jiao* Fire Channel

Figure 12

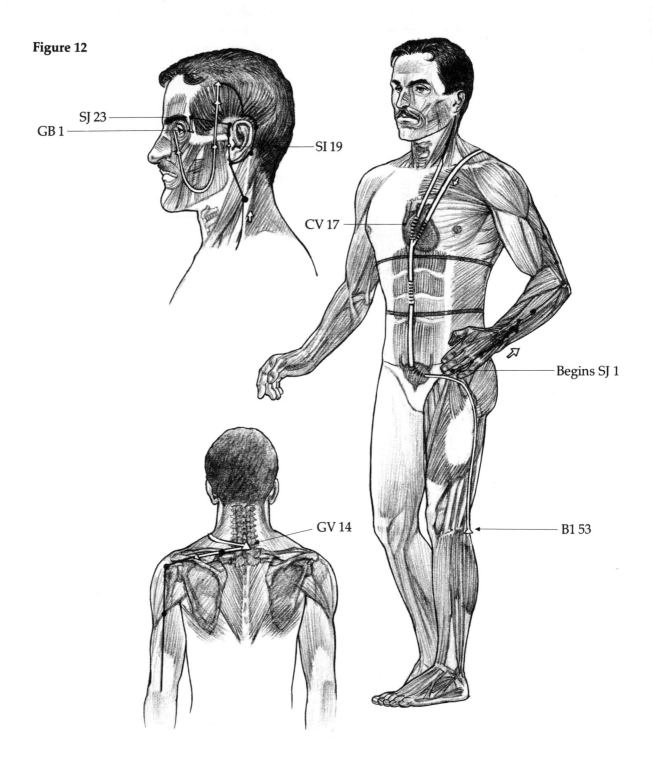

SJ 23

GB 1

SI 19

CV 17

Begins SJ 1

GV 14

B1 53

ARM LESSER YANG
SAN JIAO
FIRE CHANNEL

SUPERFICIAL—This channel originates on the ulnar nail root of the fourth digit and proceeds between the fourth and fifth metacarpal bones on the dorsum of the hand, ascending the posterior forearm between the ulna and the radius. It continues upward across the olecranon along the lateral aspect of the upper arm, passing between the lateral and long heads of the triceps, to the shoulder region. Here it intersects the Small Intestine Channel at SI 12, meets Governing Vessel Channel at GV 14, passes through GB 21, and then enters into the supraclavicular fossa. From here the channel descends DEEP into the chest region, to CV 17, where it divides into ascending and descending branches. The descending branch communicates first with the pericardium, and then descends through the diaphragm to the abdomen, linking successively with the upper, middle, and lower burners of the San Jiao. The ascending branch from CV 17 emerges (SUPERFICIAL) at the supraclavicular fossa. The channel runs up the neck to the posterior border of the ear, intersecting with Gall Bladder at GB 6 and GB 4 on the forehead, before winding downward across the cheek, through SI 18, to terminate below the eye in the infraorbital ridge. Another branch separates behind the ear and enters DEEP in the ear. It then emerges (SUPERFICIAL) in front of the ear, where it intersects the Small Intestine Channel at SI 19, crosses in front of the Gall Bladder Channel at GB 3, and traverses the cheek to terminate at the outer canthus at point SJ 23. This branch continues to connect with Gall Bladder at GB 1, also at the outer canthus. A separate branch moves from the bladder channel at the lateral popliteal fossa to connect first with the bladder organ, and then with the lower, middle, and upper burners.

LEG LESSER YANG *GALL BLADDER* WOOD CHANNEL

SUPERFICIAL—The Gall Bladder Channel begins at the outer canthus of the eye. It traverses the temple region to the area slightly below the tragus of the ear and then ascends the temple to GB 4 to intersect with St 8 at the superior hairline. From here it descends to the level of the ear, where it follows a path around the ear to the base of the occiput. GB 12 can be found posterior and inferior to the mastoid process. It ascends

Leg Lesser Yang *Gall Bladder* Wood Channel

Figure 13

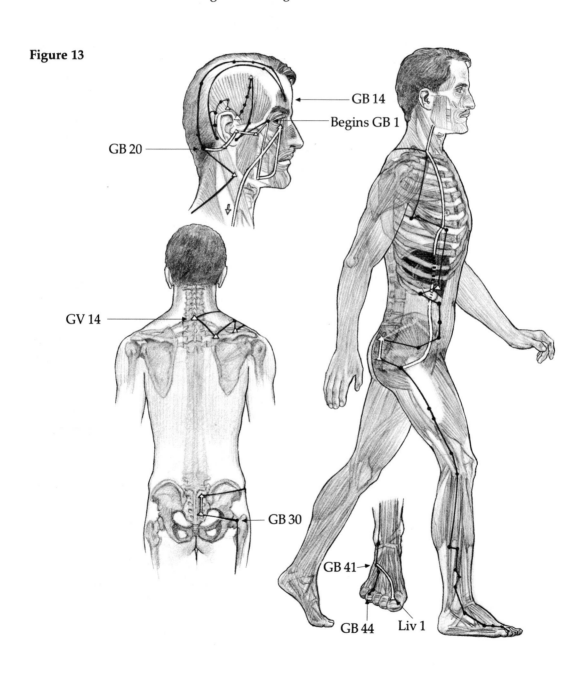

and crosses the cranium to GB 14, which can be found approximately one *tsun* above the midpoint of the eyebrow. It then moves somewhat medially before crossing and descending the cranium to GB 20, which lies in the depression between the sternocleidomastoid muscle and the lateral border of the trapezius at the base of the occiput. From GB 20 the channel intersects the Small Intestine Channel at SI 17 before descending the neck. At the top of the shoulder it turns posteromedially to intersect Governing Vessel Channel at GV 14. Finally, the channel turns antero-laterally into the supraclavicular fossa, where it divides into superficial and deep pathways. A DEEP branch originating at GB 20, behind the ear, enters into the ear. It emerges (SUPERFICIAL) in front of the ear, intersecting Small Intestine Channel at SI 19 and Stomach Channel at St 7 before reaching GB 1 at the outer canthus. A branch moves here to the jaw and then curves upward to the infraorbital region before descending again across the cheek and into the neck. Here it joins the original channel at the supraclavicular fossa, where it continues to travel in both a SUPERFICIAL and a DEEP pathway. From the supraclavicular fossa, the DEEP pathway of the channel descends into the chest, crossing the diaphragm and connecting with the liver before joining its associated organ, the gall bladder. It continues along the inside of the thorax before reaching the inguinal region of the lower abdomen. It winds around the genitalia and emerges (SUPERFICIAL) at the hip at point GB 30. The SUPERFICIAL pathway of the channel moves from the supraclavicular fossa anterior to the axilla along the lateral aspect of the chest. It passes through the Liver Channel at Liv 13 before passing through the free ends of the floating ribs. It turns posteriorly toward the sacral region, intersecting Bladder Channel on the sacrum. It passes through GB 30, joining with the DEEP pathway, and from here passes into the hip joint. It descends along the lateral aspect of the thigh to the knee. The channel continues to descend just anterior to the fibula, to the lateral malleolus. It crosses anterior to the lateral malleolus and traverses the dorsum of the foot, moving between the fourth and fifth metatarsals before terminating at GB 44 on the lateral nail root of the fourth digit. A DEEP branch separates from GB 41 and runs between the first and second metatarsals to the great toe, where it communicates with Liver Channel at Liv 1.

Leg Absolute Yin *Liver* Wood Channel

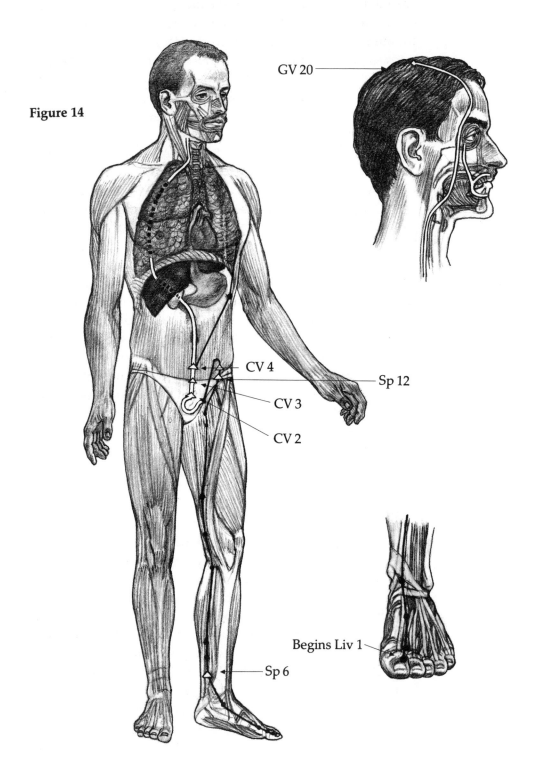

Figure 14

GV 20

CV 4

Sp 12

CV 3

CV 2

Begins Liv 1

Sp 6

LEG ABSOLUTE YIN *LIVER* WOOD CHANNEL

SUPERFICIAL—This channel begins on the dorsum of the foot at the lateral nail root of the great toe. Passing over the dorsum, it moves anterior to the medial malleolus before ascending the lower leg. It meets with the Kidney and Spleen Channels at Sp 6. It ascends the medial aspect of the leg and thigh. The channel moves from Liv 10 and 11 at the groin to spleen at Sp 12 and 13, and then to Liv 12 before descending to encircle the genitalia. It enters into the abdomen and connects with Conception Vessel Channel at CV 2, 3, and 4. Here the channel splits into superficial and deep branches. The SUPERFICIAL branch continues from CV 4 to Liv 13 at the eleventh floating rib, and then to Liv 14 at the intercostal space between the sixth and the seventh ribs. The DEEP branch ascends from the CV 4 area, encircles the stomach, and then enters into its pertaining organ, the liver, and its associated organ, the gall bladder. From here the channel continues up through the diaphragm and costal region, traverses the neck posterior to the pharynx, and enters the nasopharynx, connecting with the tissues surrounding the eye. Finally, the channel ascends across the forehead and meets with the Governing Vessel Channel at GV 20, at the vertex. A branch separates below the eye, descends into the cheek, and encircles the inside of the lips. A DEEP branch from the liver crosses the diaphragm and connects with the lungs and the Lung Channel.

Governing Vessel

Figure 15

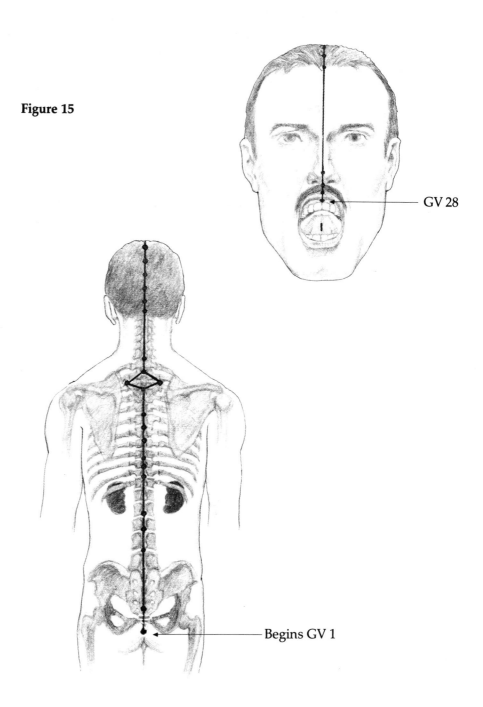

GV 28

Begins GV 1

Extraordinary Channels

GOVERNING VESSEL   The Governing Vessel is the confluence of all Yang Vessels, and there are four primary pathways through which it moves. It is illustrated in Figure 15.

1. The Governing Vessel originates at the perineum. It ascends along the spine to GV 16 at the nape of the neck. It enters into the brain, ascends to the vertex, and follows the midline of the forehead across the bridge of the nose, terminating at the labial frenum at point GV 28.[14]

2. This pathway originates in the pelvic region. It descends to the genitals and perineum and passes through the tip of the coccyx. Here it passes into the gluteal region, where it intersects the Kidney and Bladder Channels before returning to the spinal column, where it joins the kidneys.

3. The origin of the third pathway is at the same point as the Bladder Channel in the inner canthus. Two bilateral branches ascend across the forehead and converge at the vertex, where the channel enters the brain, emerging at the lower end of the nape of the neck. The channel divides again into two branches, which descend along opposite sides of the spine to the waist. Here the pathways join with the kidneys.

4. This pathway arises in the lower abdomen and ascends across the navel. It passes through the heart and enters the trachea. Continuing an upward course, the channel crosses the cheek and encircles the mouth before terminating at a point below the middle of each eye.

CONCEPTION VESSEL   There are two pathways through which this energy moves. It is illustrated in Figure 16.

1. The Conception Vessel Channel arises in the lower abdomen below point 3. It ascends along the midline of the abdomen and chest, crosses the throat and jaw, and finally winds around the mouth, terminating in the region of the eye, where this pathway intersects with ST 1 and ST 4.

2. This pathway arises in the pelvic cavity. It enters the spine and ascends along the back.

Conception Vessel

Figure 16

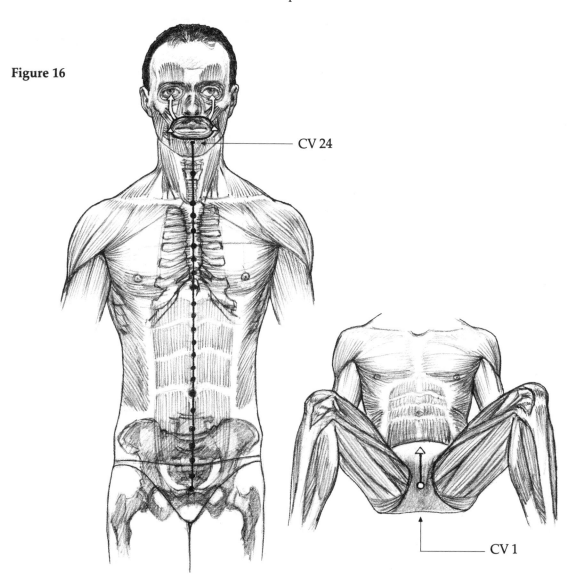

CV 24

CV 1

The Tendino-Muscle Channels

ARM GREAT YIN
TENDINO-MUSCLE
CHANNEL
(PERTAINING ORGAN—
LUNG)

This channel begins on the palmar surface of the thumb and then ascends over the radial aspect of the wrist to connect at the elbow. It continues upward over the anterior arm and enters the chest cavity above the axilla. It emerges at the clavicle and there connects at the front of the shoulder and at the clavicle. Below, it connects with the lungs and spreads over the diaphragm, finally connecting to the lower ribs.

Musculature (through which the T-M channel passes)— Opponens pollicis, abductor pollicis brevis, flexor pollicis, brachioradialis, pronator teres, biceps brachii, deltoid, pectoralis major, internal and external intercostals, diaphragm.

Arm Great Yin Tendino-Muscle Channel
(pertaining organ—Lung)

Figure 17

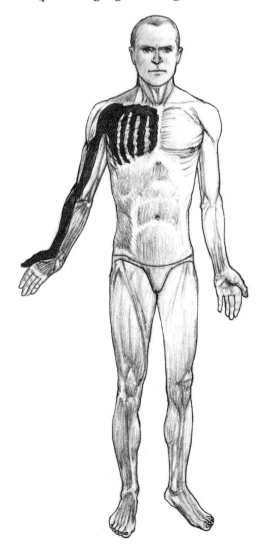

ARM BRIGHT YANG
TENDINO-MUSCLE
CHANNEL
(PERTAINING ORGAN—
COLON)

This channel begins on the dorsal tip of the index finger and moves upward to connect at the wrist. It continues over the postero-lateral forearm, narrowing at the elbow, where it connects and then continues upward, broadening as it connects to and then passes over the shoulder. The main branch passes over the top of the head and connects at the mandible on the opposite side. A branch from the shoulder spreads over the scapula and connects at the spine. A branch from the area of the union of the neck and jaw passes to the side of the nose.

Musculature   Extensor carpi radialis longus, extensor digitorum, lateral head of the triceps, deltoid, trapezius (upper and lower), infrahyoid muscles, suprahyoid muscles, scalenus, platysma, masseter (bilateral), temporalis (bilateral).

Arm Bright Yang Tendino-Muscle Channel
(pertaining organ—Colon)

Figure 18

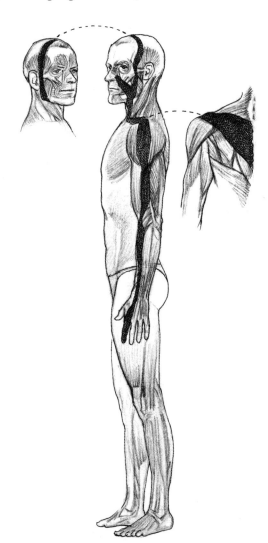

LEG BRIGHT YANG TENDINO-MUSCLE CHANNEL (PERTAINING ORGAN— STOMACH)

This channel arises at the second, third, and fourth toes, passing over the dorsum of the foot, and moves up along the lateral aspect of the tibia to the knee. The main branch continues up the antero-lateral aspect of the thigh to connect at the genital region and below the navel. It continues broadly along the antero-lateral abdomen and chest to connect at the clavicle. It moves up the side of the neck and around the mouth, finally connecting to the side of the nose. It continues up to form a muscular net around the eye with the Bladder Tendino-Muscle Channel. A branch digresses from the jaw to connect in front of the ear. Another branch arises in front of the ankle and travels more laterally up the leg to the knee. It continues to move up the lateral thigh, crossing the Gall Bladder T-M Channel to connect with the spine.

Musculature Extensor digitorum longus, tibialis anterior, vastas lateralis, rectus femoris, portions of the tensor facial lata, latissimus dorsi, transversus abdominus, rectus abdominus, platysma, jaw and facial muscles.

Figure 19

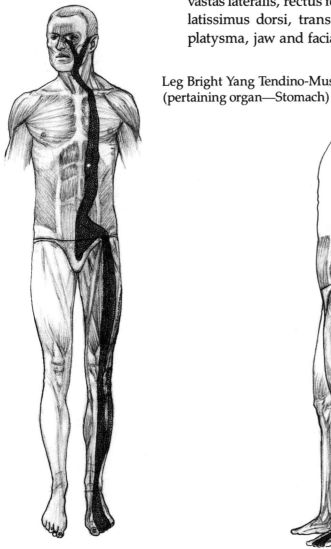

Leg Bright Yang Tendino-Muscle Channel
(pertaining organ—Stomach)

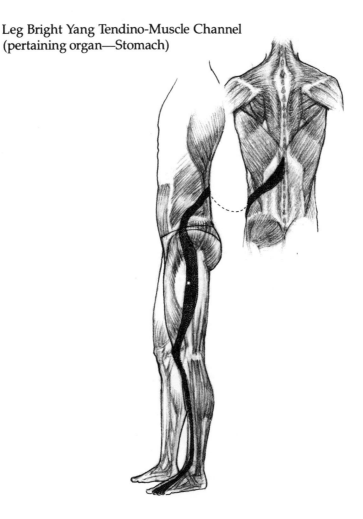

LEG GREAT YIN
TENDINO-MUSCLE
CHANNEL
(PERTAINING ORGAN—
SPLEEN)

This channel begins at the medial edge of the great toe and ascends anterior to the medial malleolus. It continues in a rather narrow path up the leg to connect at the medial condyle of the tibia. It continues in the same narrow path up the medial thigh and then to the anterior superior iliac spine. It enters the body below the navel and, moving up, curves deep inside, spreading over the ribs and connecting to the spinal column.

Musculature   Extensor hallucis, tibialis anterior, soleus, gastrocnemius, rectus femoris, sartorius, vastas medialis, transversus abdominus, internal intercostals, anterior spinal muscles.

Leg Great Yin Tendino-Muscle Channel
(pertaining organ—Spleen)

Figure 20

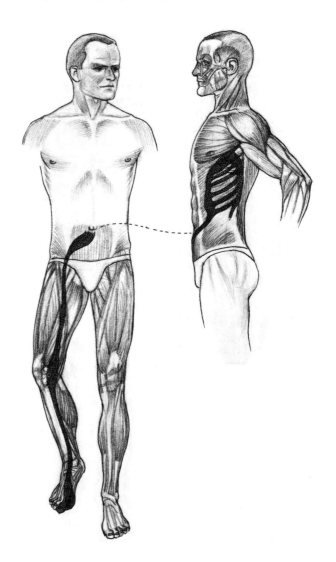

ARM LESSER YIN
TENDINO-MUSCLE
CHANNEL
(PERTAINING ORGAN—
HEART)

This channel starts on the medial aspect of the little finger and proceeds along the antero-medial aspect of the arm to the elbow. It then continues at the extreme antero-medial aspect of the upper arm to the axilla, where it enters the chest cavity. It crosses the Arm Great Yin Lung T-M and connects in the chest. A branch descends across the diaphragm and connects with the umbilicus.

Musculature   Flexor carpi ulnaris, palmaris longus, pronator teres, biceps brachii, brachial triceps, pectoralis, internal intercostals, diaphragm.

Arm Lesser Yin Tendino-Muscle Channel
(pertaining organ—Heart)

Figure 21

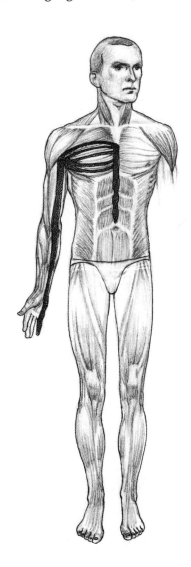

ARM GREAT YANG
TENDINO-MUSCLE
CHANNEL
(PERTAINING ORGAN—
SMALL INTESTINE)

This channel begins on the dorsal tip of the little finger and ascends along the edge of the hand to connect at the medial condyle of the elbow. It continues up the postero-medial arm to connect at the axilla, from which a branch spreads over and surrounds the scapula. From there a branch travels up the neck anterior to the Leg Great Yang Bladder Channel to connect behind the ear. A branch enters directly into the ear and emerges again at the apex of the ear, then descends along the cheek to connect at the mandible. It then curves upward to connect first at the outer canthus and then at the temple. A branch separates at the mandible and ascends around the teeth, then reconnects at the outer canthus and the temple.

Musculature   Abductor digiti minimi, extensor carpi ulnaris, extensor digiti minimi, triceps, deltoid, supraspinatus, infraspinatus, subscapularis, teres minor, teres major, trapezius, levator scapulae, rhomboids, masseter, temporalis.

Arm Great Yang Tendino-Muscle Channel
(pertaining organ—Small Intestine)

Figure 22

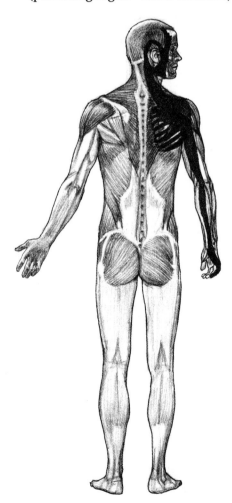

LEG GREAT YANG
TENDINO-MUSCLE
CHANNEL
(PERTAINING ORGAN—
URINARY BLADDER)

This channel arises on the lateral side of the little toe and continues upward, passing posterior to the lateral malleolus, and then connects at the knee. According to Mrs. Sohn, this branch continues up the outer edge of the leg and unites with the other leg branches at the base of the gluteus maximus. Another branch extends behind the malleolus and passes over the heel and up to the lateral edge of the popliteal fossa. A third branch separates from the second at the head of the gastrocnemius muscle and then continues up to the medial edge of the popliteal fossa. Both branches continue upward and meet the other leg branch at the gluteus. The united branches continue over the buttock and along the spine to connect at the occiput and then continue over the head to the nose. A branch from the spinal area passes under the armpit and over the chest and neck and then unites at the occiput. Another higher branch moves toward and terminates at the tip of the shoulder. A third branch separates at the level of the first

Leg Great Yang Tendino-Muscle Channel
(pertaining organ—Urinary Bladder)

Figure 23

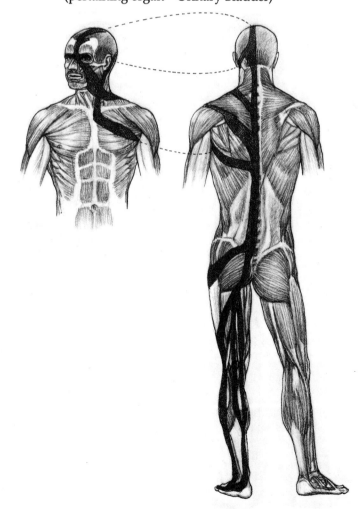

thoracic vertebra, moves up the neck and over the face to connect with the main branch coming over the head, and disperses in a web around the eye. A branch travels from the nape of the neck to the base of the tongue. Theoretical knowledge has lost the branch that moves from the spine at the waist down to the lateral margin of the hip.

Musculature   Abductor digiti minimi, flexor hallicus longus, gastrocnemius, soleus, tibialis anterior (lateral branch only), peroneus longus and brevis, semitendinosus, semimembranosus, biceps femoris, gluteus maximus, gluteus medius, erector spinae, latissimus dorsi, trapezius, galea aponeurotica (occipital and frontalis), pectoralis major, sternocleidomastoid, facial musculature.

LEG LESSER YIN TENDINO-MUSCLE CHANNEL (PERTAINING ORGAN— KIDNEY)

This channel arises on the plantar surface of the foot behind the small toe. It passes behind the medial malleolus and continues up the medial lower leg to unite at the knee. It travels in a slightly broader path up the postero-medial thigh and then over the lower abdomen quite close to the genital region. It enters the body below the navel and, moving upward, curves deep inside, moving along the side of the anterior spine to the nape of the neck. Here it unites with the occiput and connects to the Great Yang Tendino-Muscle Channel.

Musculature   Flexor digitorum brevis, tibialis anterior, tibialis posterior, flexor digitorum longus, soleus, sartorius, vastas medialis, adductor magnus, gracilis, lower abdominals, psoas major and minor, and deeper erector spinae groups of the anterior spine.

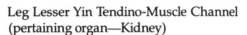

Leg Lesser Yin Tendino-Muscle Channel
(pertaining organ—Kidney)

Figure 24

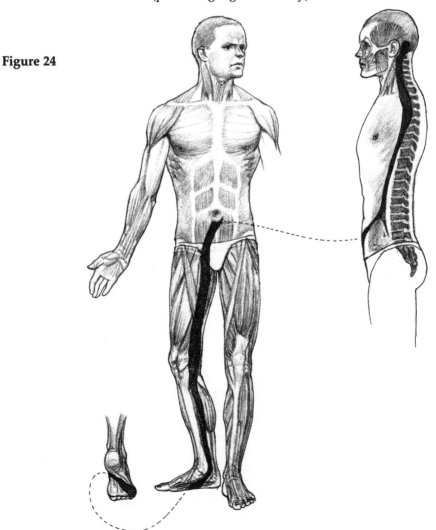

ARM ABSOLUTE YIN
TENDINO-MUSCLE
CHANNEL
(PERTAINING ORGAN—
HEART ENVELOPE)

The channel begins at the end of the middle finger on the palmar surface and continues up the antero-lateral forearm. It widens over the upper antero-medial arm and connects below the axilla. It spreads down over the ribs, front and back. A branch enters the chest below the axilla and spreads over the chest, connecting at the diaphragm.

Musculature Palmaris longus, flexor carpi radialis, biceps brachii, pectoralis, external intercostals, internal intercostals, diaphragm.

Arm Absolute Yin Tendino-Muscle Channel
(pertaining organ—Heart Envelope)

Figure 25

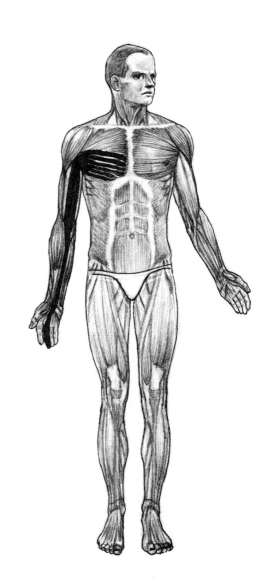

ARM LESSER YANG
TENDINO-MUSCLE
CHANNEL
(PERTAINING ORGAN—
SAN JIAO)

This channel begins at the tip of the fourth finger and travels up the dorsum of the hand to connect at the wrist. It continues up the middle of the posterior forearm and connects at the olecranon of the elbow. It then continues up the arm and over the shoulder to the neck, where it connects to the Arm Great Yang Small Intestine. A branch from the corner of the mandible passes around the neck to connect at the base of the tongue. Another branch moves upward anterior to the ear, connects at the outer canthus, and then continues over the temple to connect at the side of the forehead.

Musculature Extensor digitorum, triceps brachii, deltoid, sternocleidomastoid, hyoid group, masseter, temporalis.

Arm Lesser Yang Tendino-Muscle Channel
(pertaining organ—San Jiao)

Figure 26

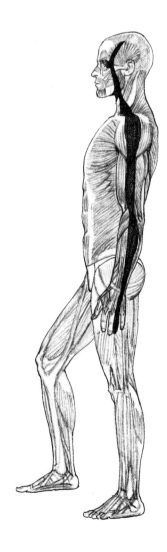

LEG LESSER YANG
TENDINO-MUSCLE
CHANNEL
(PERTAINING ORGAN—
GALL BLADDER)

The channel begins at the fourth toe and connects to the lateral malleolus. It then travels up the antero-lateral leg to connect at the side of the knee. A branch from the top of the fibula continues up the thigh, widening as it approaches the hip. A small branch breaks off above the knee and travels anterior to the main stomach channel. A branch separates from the main branch at the level of the acetabulum and moves posteriorly over the buttock to connect with the sacrum. The main branch continues up to pass in front of the axilla. A branch departs at the point of connection with the ribs and moves over the chest to reunite with the main branch at the level of the shoulder. It continues up behind the ear and connects at the temple and to its bilateral counterpart at the vertex. A branch descends from the temple, crosses the cheek, and finally connects with the bridge of the nose. A branch separates on the cheek and connects to the outer canthus.

Musculature   Extensor digitorum, peroneus longus, peroneus brevis, tibialis anterior, tensor fascia latae, ilio-tibial tract, gluteus maximus, serratus anterior, pectoralis, transversus abdominis, deltoid, trapezius, sternocleidomastoid, epicranius, facial muscles, temporalis.

Figure 27   Leg Lesser Yang Tendino-Muscle Channel (pertaining organ—Gall Bladder)

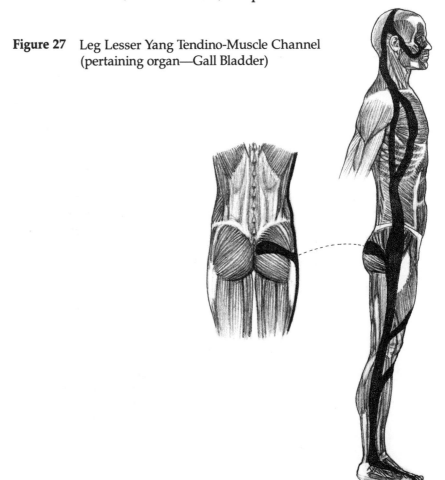

LEG ABSOLUTE YIN
TENDINO-MUSCLE
CHANNEL
(PERTAINING ORGAN—
LIVER)

The channel begins on the dorsum of the foot at the great toe and passes anterior to the medial malleolus before continuing up along the medial tibia to connect at the knee. It then continues up the thigh, passing above the genitals. It enters the body below the navel and connects to several other Tendino-Muscle Channels.

Musculature   Extensor hallucis, tibialis anterior, gastrocnemius, gracilis, adductor magnus, vastus medialis, rectus abdominis.

Leg Absolute Yin Tendino-Muscle Channel
(pertaining organ—Liver)

Figure 28

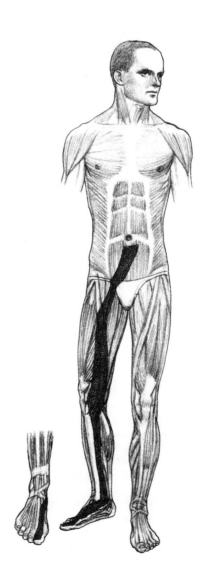

Cutaneous Regions—Front View

Figure 29

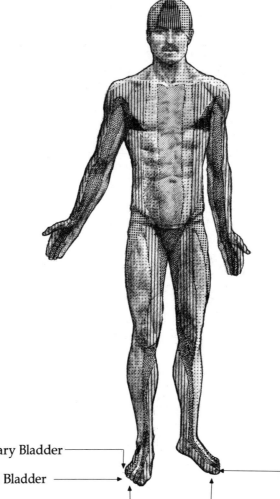

Note: Great Yang Urinary Bladder

Note: Lesser Yang Gall Bladder

Note: Bright Yang Stomach

Note: Absolute Yin Liver

Note: Great Yin Spleen

Legend

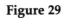	Great Yin: Arm Lung / Leg Spleen		Bright Yang: Arm Colon / Leg Stomach
	Lesser Yang: Arm San Jiao / Leg Gall Bladder		Great Yang: Leg Urinary Bladder / Arm Small Intestine
	Absolute Yin: Arm Heart Envelope / Leg Liver		Lesser Yin: Arm Heart / Leg Kidney

Cutaneous Regions—Back View

Figure 30

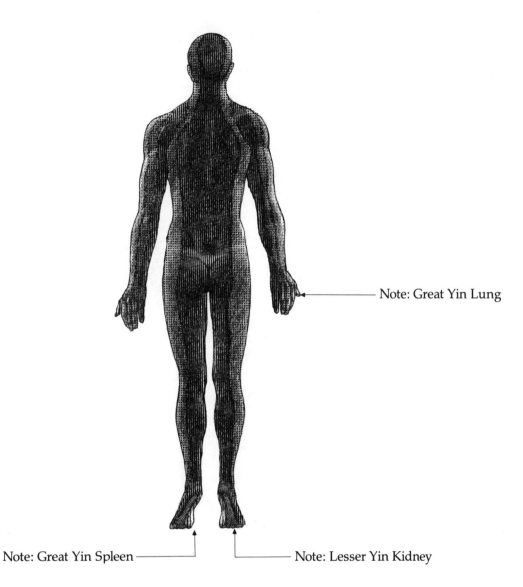

— Note: Great Yin Lung

Note: Great Yin Spleen ——————   ———— Note: Lesser Yin Kidney

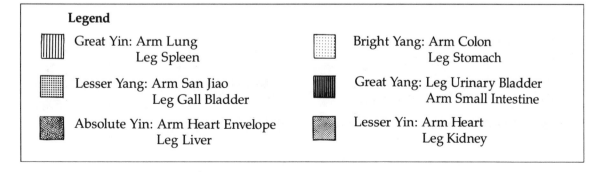

Legend

Great Yin:	Arm Lung Leg Spleen	Bright Yang:	Arm Colon Leg Stomach
Lesser Yang:	Arm San Jiao Leg Gall Bladder	Great Yang:	Leg Urinary Bladder Arm Small Intestine
Absolute Yin:	Arm Heart Envelope Leg Liver	Lesser Yin:	Arm Heart Leg Kidney

Cutaneous Regions—Side View

Figure 31

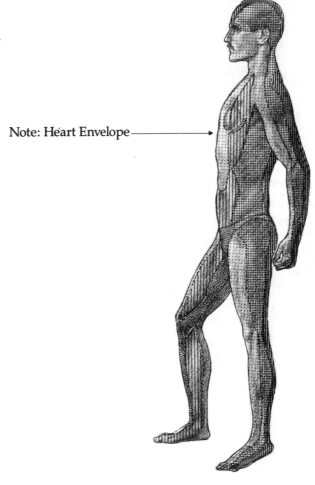

Note: Heart Envelope ⎯⎯⎯⎯⎯⎯⎯→

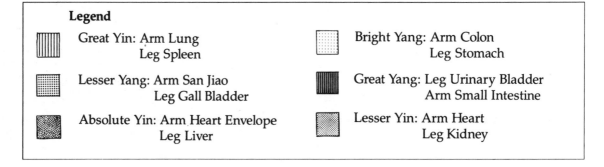

Legend

Great Yin: Arm Lung Leg Spleen		Bright Yang: Arm Colon Leg Stomach	
Lesser Yang: Arm San Jiao Leg Gall Bladder		Great Yang: Leg Urinary Bladder Arm Small Intestine	
Absolute Yin: Arm Heart Envelope Leg Liver		Lesser Yin: Arm Heart Leg Kidney	

Endnotes   [1] It may be suggested that acupuncture caused a sensitization of the parotid gland which then transmitted the vibratory energy to the left auditory nerve. The difference in the quality and intensity of the energy was then interpreted by the brain as a signal from the damaged right auditory nerve. If this is the case, it again shows the primacy of function over structure, and we are pleased that structure is so accommodating to function that it changes for the sake of function.

[2] Manfred Porket, *The Essentials of Chinese Diagnostics* (Zurich: Acta Medicinae Sinensis, Chinese Medicine Publications, Ltd., 1983), pp. 1–15.

[3] This demonstrates why the Diminishing Yin stage cannot be the middle stage of Yin. Since Yin must continue to grow into the final stage and then rapidly decline, only the Yin which diminishes can be at that final stage. And since the middle stage is still growing into the final stage, Diminishing Yin cannot be the middle stage, as it is contrary in its growth pattern.

[4] The discussion that follows will became much clearer after the section on the function and relationships of the Organs and Channels has been read. Several ideas must be taken without explanation at this time, as they are only illustrative, and the reader is not expected to learn to use them, but to try to see the rational relationships that are expressed.

[5] The Lung is considered to be one organ if you consider the single-source bronchus as branching into two main sections.

[6] Remember that the Pancreas function is considered part of the orb of influence of the Spleen in Chinese medicine.

[7] Reinhold Voll, M.D., *Topographic Positions of the Measurement Points in Electro Acupuncture*, translated and fully revised by Hartwig Schuldt, M.D., M.S. (Velzen: Medizinisch Literarische Verlagsgesellschaft, 1977).

[8] *Acupuncture: A Comprehensive Text.* Shanghai College of Traditional Medicine. Translated and edited by John O'Connor and Dan Bensky, Seattle: Eastland Press, 1974.

[9] It is interesting to note that East Indian yogis also see the brain, essence, and sperm as interconnected. Jing Qi is broadly essence or Vital Qi, and, narrowly, semen. Indian yogis, practicing celibacy, state that Ojas (sperm) is saved and carried to the brain during pranayama, where it is transformed into spiritual energy for circulation in the central channel. It is probable that this concept relates to cerebrospinal fluid.

[10] The channel here termed Heart Envelope is frequently found in literature under various other names, including Pericardium, Circulation-Sex, and Heart Constrictor. San Jiao is frequently termed Triple Heater, Triple Burner, and Three Heaters. The reasons for the existence of these various terms are discussed in the section "Comments on the Names of the Pathways of Qi." The terms Heart Envelope and San Jiao are used throughout the text.

[11] There is Fire in the Liver and Kidney as well as in the four organ channels that are assigned to the Fire phase. Various events can affect the Liver so that its Fire can become excess, both through the overactivity of its Son and the burning of the Liver Wood. Fire tends to rise, and this Liver Fire Rising will affect the eyes and head, in particular, as the Liver opens into the eyes.

[12] It should be noted here that an important text, *Acupuncture: A Comprehensive Text* (Shanghai College of Traditional Medicine, translated and edited by John O'Connor and Dan Bensky. Seattle: Eastland Press, 1974, p. 39) describes Ancestral Qi as being formed from the Qi of Air and the Nourishing Qi (which we have called the Qi of Grain) combining in the chest, and then acting as the driving *qi* of the channels. Most authorities agree that it is the Yuan Qi of the Kidneys that drives the other energies, including Blood, through the channels and blood vessels. We have indicated that the Ancestral Qi created in the chest can, under the appropriate conditions, be used to replenish the Yuan Qi.

[13] The same establishment ostracized Semmelweis because he blamed allopathic physicians for the spread of puerperal fever and death from complications of childbirth of 3 to 25 percent of hospitalized women, as a result of disease organisms spread by physicians who performed operations and dissections one after another without washing their hands.

[14] Governing Vessel 28, at the labial frenum, is the union point of the Conception Vessel and the Governing Vessel.

PART THREE

The Practice

———————————————

CHAPTER SIX
The Hand

"My fingers are my eyes and ears."
MRS. TINA SOHN

KINESTHETIC awareness and physical development are essential in the training of an Amma therapist. More essential, however, is the development of a particularly keen awareness in the hands. The hands serve a twofold purpose for the therapist. They are the sensors with which to feel, and the tools with which to work. Hands are used throughout the work day both for treating patients and for assessing their condition.

For the Amma therapist, touch is the most essential sense, and the hands are the most important organs of this sense. They are, without doubt, the most highly evolved organs for the performance of even the most subtle manipulative task. Although the sense of touch is often connected to the hands, and not the skin surface generally, the hands are the least developed of our sensory organs. Used well, however, the hands serve as a primary information-gathering device. They can assess important data relative to the patient's condition, differentiating, for example, throughout the body, variations in muscular tonus, temperature, and skin quality. With long and serious practice and carefully channelled attention, increasingly more subtle signals can be received from the patient's body through the hands. The trained hands of an Amma therapist can palpate and interpret qualities of vascular activity and its disturbances, respiratory rhythms and their anomalies, cerebrospinal rhythmic pulsation and its disturbances, and even the patterns of flow and disturbances of bioenergy.

If you wish to use your hands to sense the condition of the patient on subtle and significant levels, and not to follow mechanically a prearranged series of motions, you must mold your hands into tools to serve your will. You must make them *acutely sensitive.* This is accomplished through constant attention, through placing awareness into the hands, learning to *feel intentionally* with them. You feel objects all day long—the pen with which you write, the keys on the typewriter, the glass from which you drink, the water with which you wash. Yet *most* of what you feel goes unnoticed. You have no need to be more than superficially aware of the tactile sensations produced by the mass of objects and forces that you experience in most of the activities of life. The sensations entering through all sense organs including the hands are monitored and filtered by the brain so that only those things needing "special handling" by the conscious elements, or those things that are awaited intentionally by those same conscious elements, are allowed to enter beyond peripheral awareness. Thus, the first step in creating these tools, these sensors, is to pay attention to them.

Each area of the hand—the palm, each finger, the pad of each finger, the thumb and thenar eminence—can provide information about what is being touched. Each finger senses individually, and therefore attention must be given to each finger and each area of the hand individually. There is no limit to time or place in the process of developing the sensitivity of these tools. It does not require the manipulation of a physical body.

Your daily activities, from the moment you awaken constantly involve the use of your hands to hold, manipulate, touch, and assess a myriad of objects. You should begin to be aware of all the information available from your hands about all the objects that you touch. The different qualities of metals, woods, plastics, fabrics, and organic substances can be felt, as well as hardness, softness, roughness, and smoothness. Density, thinness, or thickness of substances are more difficult, but can be felt with the hands. Even the distinction between hard plastics and bone or ivory can be clearly felt with well-sensitized hands. They are remarkable devices. With consistent training the sense of touch can be as keen as the clearest eyesight, and can provide information of the most subtle nature to the evolved practitioner. Mrs. Sohn has said, "My fingers are my eyes and ears." The Amma therapist must seek to evolve to the same level of manual sensitivity.

The hands must be sufficiently strong and flexible to be able to consistently manifest and control the technical skill required in Amma therapy. For Amma to be the therapeutic modality it is intended to be, and not deteriorate into the "bath house rubbing" that other devolving bodywork forms have sometimes become, strength and flexibility are also essential. However, strength in the hands alone is insufficient. There must be sufficient strength in the arms, shoulders, and back as well, to deliver even pressure throughout the treatment without allowing fatigue to diminish that pressure. Inadequate strength, or strength that is manifest in spurts, is unacceptable. It results in poking and jabbing at the patient, and may be the cause of unnecessary pain. For the Amma therapist, strength is the ability to sustain a reasonable, intense level of effort for a long time without deterioration; it is the capacity for exertion and endurance sustained without deviation for the extent of at least one treatment.

Amma therapy requires sufficient strength in the upper body to guide, manage, and direct the hands and arms for the finely detailed movements involved in subtle hand and finger techniques as well as the broader movements of the hands and arms. Fine movements of the fingers are accomplished through actions of the intrinsic muscles of the hands. However, the larger, "gross" movements of the hands are accomplished by actions of the muscles of the forearms. Since the origins of many of the forearm muscles are on the humerus, actions of the forearm muscles on the hands involves some activation of the upper arm. Movement of the upper arms is a direct function of the muscles of the chest, shoulders, and back, again because of the origins and insertions of the muscles in these regions. The movement of the hands and arms, then, involves the total musculature of the upper body and is directly affected by the strength of that muscle system.

Strength in the legs, abdomen, and upper back is necessary simply to maintain an upright posture. Weakness of the torso muscles leads to fatigue, which invariably results in leaning on the hands and arms, and even on the patient, instead of using the hands as tools. A treatment lasts for approximately fifty minutes, with the therapist standing most of the time and directing pressure into the patient's body. The back and legs must be fully developed to support the body in this upright, but often forward-leaning, position and to allow the hands and arms to apply controlled pressure. The therapist must be capable of accomplishing fifty minutes of hard physical work without straining. The breath must remain even and under control. Stamina and endurance must be evolved so that the last technique of the treatment is applied with the same power and focus as the first. The therapist must be able to concentrate fully on the patient without being distracted by the aches and pains that inevitably result from inadequate or incomplete physical development. The level of strength and, therefore, physical development of the Amma therapist is equal to that required in the development of a serious athlete.

The Amma therapist's primary strength must be manifest both in and through the hands. Mrs. Sohn's hand strength is such that she can break an apple neatly in half with her hands. Strength in the hands is necessary for control of the hands. Control is the ability to guide or manage the hand for proper treatment, including guiding the hands to the appropriate points and areas of the body, maintaining the sometimes difficult positions that the hands and fingers must hold, properly maintaining the direction of force, and properly maintaining the quantity of force. Great strength must be developed in the small muscles of the hand as well as in the muscles of each finger. Each finger must move independently to hold points and control direction of applied force without losing strength or allowing the force to dissipate into the palm or other fingers. Occasionally the hands are rotated and maintained in unusual and sometimes uncomfortable positions as specific areas of the body are treated. For example, the inner canthus of the eye is treated with the lateral aspect of the tip of the pad of the fifth digit. The point must be held and manipulated. Should the hand slip, it may do injury to the eye of the patient. Development of the small muscles of the hand is required to accomplish this manipulation without danger to the patient. Strength is the root on which control grows. Both are essential in the development of the hands of the practitioner.

Relaxation of the hand and body is necessary for adequate development of both sensitivity and strength. We often mistake tension for strength. People will tighten muscles to "feel" strong, but as martial arts students soon begin to learn, as long as they "feel strong" through muscular tension, whatever strength or power they can develop is lost to the effort of the contraction. The experience is only the power of the muscular contraction. The subjective "feeling of strength" is the very thing that opposes the attempt to manifest real strength. For a practitioner of Amma, real strength lies in the ability to direct a force into another body. This force will be of greatest value when it is highly concentrated and directed. When force is contained in the maintenance of the muscle contraction, the force is lost within that muscle. Force developed through muscle contraction will not be expended at its intended location, that is, at the point of contact with the patient. During the peak of her practice at the Wholistic Health Center, Mrs. Sohn regularly treated between seventeen and twenty-three patients a day, six days a week. Remember that in Amma therapy, strength is the capacity for exertion and endurance sustained without deviation for the extent of at least one treatment.

Using the body correctly allows real force to be manifested. Proper and consistent alignment of the musculo-skeletal system provides a channel through which force can easily be developed and directed. If the alignment is maintained over a reasonable period of time, surprising degrees of stamina in consistent application of powerful force can be easily accomplished and with minimal amounts of tension and muscular contraction. Once the skeletal alignment of the body and hands are properly maintained, the attention should be directed to relaxing the musculature, with only those muscles and tendons directly involved in maintaining alignment allowed to remain in contraction. The hand is open—the fingers neither hyperextended nor curled toward the palm. The musculature is relaxed and soft, and no joint is locked (although there must be sufficient tonus in the hands to maintain an alignment between the central metacarpal and the centerline of the forearm). Energy as force will move through a relaxed muscle but will be lost in the constriction of a muscle locked in unnecessary contraction. Therefore, when the body is aligned and tension is relaxed in the muscles of the legs, buttocks, torso, chest, neck, face, arms, and hands, real strength, from the free flow of systemic energy, will be experienced.[1] At this point the practitioner can direct the force for various purposes throughout the course of an Amma treatment.

We begin with the development of muscular strength. We use this strength to develop and maintain proper musculo-skeletal alignment. Through this alignment, force can be directed while the musculature can be properly relaxed. Finally, trained and relaxed, the hands can begin to feel what is being touched. Relaxation of the hand is necessary in the development of sensitivity. A hand that is stiff with tension, that is held almost as a claw, cannot feel what is beneath the skin to differentiate even among the muscles that drape the body. When the physical strength is such that all that is necessary can be accomplished with ease during the course of a treatment, the practitioner can begin to make the more subtle efforts to evolve hand sensitivity resulting in deeper awareness. When the hand can mold to the contours of the body as it moves over the surface, and when areas and points can be manipulated with directed force while maintaining physical relaxation, *then* the mind can be directed to attending to feeling more deeply into the complex multiplicity of signals and indicators of the patient's body. Such indications as temperature changes, subtle swellings or areas of fullness, areas of weakness or strain, areas that feel "spongey" or "brittle" become gross and obvious facts next to the subtle and powerful indicators of the patient's condition available to truly sensitive hands. Your hands are your sensors as well as your tools.

Focused attention within yourself and toward your patient is the element that makes the hands into powerful and subtle sensors. Focused attention is the means by which a practitioner can learn to become delicately aware and capable of perceiving minute fluctuations in the patient's physical and emotional condition. Physical sensitivity, the awareness of the condition of the physical body through the sense of touch, begins with a tactile awareness of the tone and texture of the skin and musculature. It can lead to the ability to sense the most subtle biological activities including respiratory rhythms, circulatory functioning, and qualities of the cerebrospinal rhythmic pulsations. Sensitivity allows the practitioner to become aware of the physical manifestation of a patient's emotional experience. It provides the ability to become aware of emotional states as they are experienced by the patient. Ultimately it provides the ability to become aware of the bioenergy system. There is a world of experience available to the touch of a practitioner with developed sensitivity which is never available to others. Very few are born with the gift of extreme sensitivity. For those who are not, focused attention is the means through which it can be developed.

The practice of palpation is used as an exercise to develop relaxation and sensitivity in the hands. Palpation is exploration through touching the patient's body; it is examination by use of the hands. Through palpation, the superficial and deeper structures of the body are experienced, and the student of Amma arrives at a broader understanding of the structure of the human body. Skin qualities, muscle shapes and qualities, tendon insertions, blood vessels and anastomoses, lymph vessels and nodes, are examples of a few of the multitude of parts experienced through attentive and directed practice of palpation. This practice begins with understanding through formal study the physical structure and its functions. Surface anatomy, general anatomy, and detailed myology must be studied carefully and completely to produce a thorough understanding of the musculo-skeletal system. The size, shape, and purpose of the structures within the skeletal system must be understood, as well as the structure and operation of the various joints. The aspiring Amma therapist must become equally familiar with the muscular system, learning the size, shape and actions, fiber directions, enervation, and vascularization of each of the many muscles of the body. This formal study must be enlivened by study of the therapist's own body.

Begin the practice of palpation by touching your body. Use your entire hand, and gently stroke over the surface of an area of your body. Try to sense its form and structure with your hand. Become aware of each part of your hand and what is felt in each part as you move your hand over your limb or torso. If you feel that one or another part of the hand is not in contact with the muscle, soften the hand. Allow it to mold to the body's contours. The form of the hand will change as it moves from one area of the body to another since the contours of the body change. Allow your hand to assume the contours of the surface over which it moves. Your hand must be constantly corrected to retain maximum relaxation. Use a gentle touch to lightly contact the surface of the body. There is no need to apply pressure; simply feel the texture of the skin and the configuration of the surface musculature. Feel the interstices between the muscles. Feel the tendons and the superficial blood vessels. Discern the form of the surface muscles. Start at the origin and follow each muscle to its insertion, attending to the size and shape of the muscle as well as its qualities like fullness or emptiness, spasm or flaccidity. Feel for temperature variations and local spasms throughout the area being palpated. Look at what is being palpated and visualize the form of the muscle, as well as its placement and action. Combine your cognitive awareness with your sensory experience and you will broaden your understanding of the physical form.

When you can comfortably palpate the surface and sense the necessary configurations and differentiations, you should increase the depth of palpation and try to feel the skeletal structure. This new practice should encompass the face, skull, and posterior neck, and continue to the rib cage, the shoulders, the legs, arms, hands, and feet. First you will become aware of the basic structure of the bones. You must try to become aware of the small hollows, ridges, and hairline cracks on the surface of the bones. Use the same technique of combining cognitive awareness with sensory experience. As you continually focus your mind to attend to what you are feeling your experience of the body will change dramatically. Your level of skill in palpation will increase and you will be on your way to developing your hands into the sensors and the tools that you need to become a skilled practitioner of this art.

Since balance is an essential aspect of the development of an Amma therapist, work with both hands, so that both hands may be equal in strength and sensitivity. Each person has a dominant hand: the hand used to write. The imbalance between the dominant and nondominant hands can be corrected by using the nondominant hand to *replace* the dominant hand in simple daily activities such as brushing the teeth, using eating utensils, buttoning a shirt, closing a lid on a jar, or reaching for a glass of water. Learning to write with the nondominant hand develops the finer muscles of the hand and arm and cultivates fine coordination. By requiring the nondominant hand to do these tasks, daily activities become a major exercise for developing balance in the Amma therapist.

The ever greater and finer development of the hands on each level of ability requires directed attention, persistent practice, and constant correction. The result is the production of a pair of finely tuned instruments. As they are honed, these instruments will begin to produce wonderful experiences. They will be tools of great value, and sensors of unimagined sensitivity, and will serve you well in your work as an Amma therapist.

An Anatomical Description

In our discussion of the various hand techniques that are used in Amma therapy you are directed to use certain areas of the hand. The following is a detailed description of the parts of the hand as this relates to the various techniques and exercises described in subsequent parts of this text:

> The pad of the finger is the soft fleshy area of the most distal aspect of the digit. This provides a soft, but firm area for the application of pressure. The pads of the fingers are used on many areas of the body in a variety of technique forms.

> The free edge of the finger is the region that lies between the apex of the pad of the digit and the tip of the digit. It is the fleshy area that overlies the head of the distal phalange of each digit. This is the area of the finger that is used in various hand exercises, as well as in a greater portion of the manipulations applied using circular digital pressure and direct pressure techniques.

> The palmar aspect of the finger is the area that extends from the most distal aspect of the finger to the surface of the palm that covers the metacarpophalangeal joint. The fingers are held together as a unit in a relaxed manner, creating a plane which contacts the body. This area of the hand is used on the larger muscle groups of the body.

The palm is the area which includes the thenar and hypothenar regions and extends from the base of the fingers to the wrist. It provides a large area which can be used as a flat surface or can create a drawing motion, or adhering quality. An embracing motion is often used on the extremities and the shoulders. The flat palm can be used along the lower back and hip area and when the patient is very sensitive.

The palm-heel area of the hand is the area at the proximal aspect of the palm covering the carpal bones. It can be used to manipulate large areas, such as the base of the buttocks.

The thumb is used frequently during the course of the Amma treatment. The arch of the thumb is the area covering and extending to either side of the most distal joint. The thenar region, the fleshy base of the thumb, is its guiding force. The thumb is often used in the application of direct pressure, circular pressure, and stroking techniques.

The blade of the hand, or the ulnar aspect of the hand, extends from the distal aspect of the small finger along the edge of the fifth metacarpal to the wrist on the ulnar side of the hand. This is used in the chopping technique.

Care of the Hands

Since the hands are the sensors with which you gather information and the tools with which Amma is administered, it is important that they are cared for properly. A few basic rules should be followed to insure proper care and appearance of your hands.

1. Protect your hands with gloves when working in the house or garden or whenever you do any type of work that could cause your hands to become chapped, callused, blistered, or cut.

2. During colder weather use a natural hand lotion or cream to protect your hands from drying or cracking.

3. Keep your nails trimmed short, using a nail file or emery board to avoid sharp edges. Because of the type of pressure techniques that are applied during the administration of Amma, long nails may leave marks, bruises, or cuts on your patient.

4. Do not bite your nails or the skin at the edges of the nails. You must recognize that nail-biting is a nervous habit that stems from your own emotional distress. Part of becoming a therapist is an awareness and control of your own emotional environment.

5. Do not cut your cuticles. This can lead to infection. You may push them back using an orange stick.

6. Do not use nail polishes of any kind. Polishes chip and crack causing your hands to become unsightly.

7. After exercising your hands place them under alternating hot and cold running water. Close and open your hands while under the water to help relax them.

8. Do not wear rings or bracelets while treating patients, only a lightweight watch if necessary.

9. Wash your hands with cold water after treating each patient. This helps to prevent the assimilation of energies taken in from the patient you have treated. If there is a feeling of discomfort in the hands and especially in the arms after treating ill patients, shake your hands, as you would shake a thermometer, to release the energy from your own body.

10. If needed, use a natural lotion or hand cream after washing your hands to maintain a smooth hand surface.

Endnotes   [1] This alignment is the basic practice of T'ai Chi Chuan, which is required as part of the curriculum of the New Center for Wholistic Health Education and Research. It was inconceivable for a person to be an herbalist or acupuncturist in ancient China without being a master of T'ai Chi Chuan. We hope to introduce this practice in modern America, and thereby revitalize the health care system of the modern world.

CHAPTER SEVEN
Hand Exercises

THIS series of hand exercises should be practiced daily to develop strength, coordination, and sensitivity.

Exercises 1–5 are done while in a kneeling position on the floor. The buttocks are resting on the heels.

1. FINGER STRETCH

Place your palms flat on the floor so that the centers of your palms are flush with the floor and no spaces are evident between the floor and the perimeter of your hand, at the wrist fold, or at the webbed areas between the fingers. Elongate your fingers, stretching each finger out so that it is as long and as flat as possible. Relax your fingers. Do not allow them to bend. Keep them straight and relaxed. Hold this position for ten to fifteen seconds. Slowly withdraw your hands from the floor and shake them out. Repeat this four or five times.

This exercise will develop stretch in the fingers and palms, and begins the development of the fine muscles of the palm, which are being used to keep it flat on floor.

2. PALMAR EMBRACE

Place your palms on the floor as in Exercise 1.

Be sure that there are no spaces evident at any point around the perimeter of the hand. Focusing on the center of the palm, draw this area away from the floor making certain that the direction of force is directly upward. You will see only a slight movement of the muscles along the entire perimenter of the hand. Practically no movement will occur with the gross muscles of the hand. This is an exercise for the very fine muscles of the hand, and the mind.

There is a tendency, when doing this exercise, to draw the center of the palm upward so that only the muscles of the radial aspect of the hand are involved. This is incorrect. The ulnar aspect of the hand must also be used. In addition, there will be a tendency for the weight of your arms to be forced into the palm-heel area of your hand. Try to avoid this. Keep the weight evenly distributed throughout your hand.

After the palm is drawn upward, relax it again so that the centermost part is touching the floor. This is similar to the action of a suction cup. Repeat this motion ten to fifteen times, taking care to maintain straight, relaxed fingers. Slowly withdraw your hands from the floor and shake them out.

The purpose of this exercise is to develop the awareness of the fine muscles of the palm, as well as to strengthen them. These muscles are used in the execution of the palmar embrace technique used during the administration of the Basic Amma.

3. WRIST STRETCH   Place your palms on the floor so that the anterior aspects of the wrists are touching, and the fingertips are pointed in opposite directions. Stretch your fingers out as far as possible, making certain that there are no spaces evident between the floor and the perimeter of your hand. The elbow folds on the ventral surface of your arms will be facing away from your body. Keeping your fingers stretched, without allowing the knuckles to bend, slowly rotate your forearms so that the elbow folds are facing each other. Do not allow the palm-heel area of the hands to lift up off the floor. Do not allow your shoulders to roll forward as your rotate your forearms. Hold this position for five counts, and then slowly rotate your forearms back to the initial position. Repeat four to five times.

This exercise is instrumental in evolving stretch and flexibility in the palmar surface of the hands, the wrists, and forearms.

4. FINGERTIPS   Place your *fingertips* on the floor so that your fingers are relaxed, but extended. The palm of your hand is well up off the floor. The joints in your fingers and hands are neither flexed nor extended. Keep your hands and fingers relaxed, but straight, without bending the knuckles. Your hands take on the appearance of a smooth, curved line that extends from your fingertips to your wrist. Gradually shift your weight onto your fingertips, repeatedly checking to make sure that your fingers remain straight. The *most* distal aspect of the palmar surface of each finger, *not the pads* of the distal phalanges, is in contact with the floor. Hold this position for five counts and release. Repeat this four to five times. Withdraw your hands and shake them out.

When you are able to maintain this position without locking

or bending any of the joints in your fingers or hands, slowly lift your knees off the floor approximately two to three inches. Hold this position for five counts, release, and then repeat four to five times.

Both parts of this exercise develop proper alignment of the fingers and the strength that is necessary for adequate hand control when using digital pressure techniques.

Exercises 5–8 are done while seated either tailor fashion or in a kneeling position.

5. CROSSING FINGERS   To stretch the fingers and develop flexibility, the children's game of crossing the fingers is a good exercise. Place the fifth digit over the fourth, the fourth over the third, the third over the second. Hold this position for five to ten counts, and then slowly relax the fingers and shake out your hands.

6. ROLLING STONES   A very good, very accessible method of exercise for the hands is done with two large walnuts or stones of that approximate size. Both should fit comfortably in the palm of one hand. Exercise the fingers and hands by rolling the walnuts or stones around in the palm of the hand. A variation on this exercise is to roll and squeeze a hard rubber ball in the palm of the hand. The rolling and squeezing motion develops strength and co-ordination of the fine muscles of the hands and fingers.

7. FIST-STRETCH   In order to build strength and endurance the following exercise is recommended. Make a tight fist, closing the thumb around the fingers. From the fist position, fan your hands out, stretch-ing the palms and fingers as widely as possible. Alternate the fist position with the stretch position. Alternate fist and stretch, beginning with fifteen to twenty-five rounds. Work up to one hundred fifty to two hundred rounds. Build up slowly, without sacrificing the detail of correct fist and stretch posi-tions for each round you can accomplish.

8. ROTATING THUMBS   This exercise is used to relax the hands and develop muscle isolation of the individual muscles in the thenar region. In addition it serves to strengthen the muscles of the thenar region.

Keep the thumbs abducted and extended, keeping them straight at the interphalangeal joints. Rotate the thumbs, first in a clockwise direction and then counterclockwise. You must make certain that the rotation takes place from the *carpo-metacarpal joint*, and not the metacarpo-phalangeal joint. Begin with twenty-five rounds and work up slowly to ninety to one hundred rounds.

9. STRENGTHENING THE WRISTS

Tie one end of a cord to a one- or two-pound weight and the other end to the center of a wood dowel. Stand with the arms extended at shoulder height. Elbows must remain straight, but not locked. Hold the dowel in both hands, palms facing downward, allowing the weight to hang freely. Using the muscles of the hand only, wind the cord around the dowel, drawing the weight up to it. Once the weight is up, reverse the winding movement so that the weight is lowered toward the ground, making sure to control the descent carefully. Repeat this exercise two or three times. The same exercise may be done with the palms turned upward.

CHAPTER EIGHT
Hand Techniques

Circular Pressure

THIS is the most commonly used technique in Amma therapy. It is a combination of light pressure and circular movement at a given point. By breaking the technique down to its primary components, we can see that it involves the application of light pressure and movement in small circles at a given point on the body, moving approximately one inch from that point on a predetermined line of movement and then repeating the press-circle-move cycle. Movement is even and rhythmic, resembling that of a spiraling line. For example, manipulation of the inner arm begins at the axilla, and proceeds toward the little finger with movement proceeding in a circling motion down the inner arm. In the novice practitioner, who has yet to develop fine coordination, the circles will frequently be rather large, covering much surface area. However, in the master therapist, the size of the circle is minimal, often producing *the appearance* of movement in a straight line or in an up-and-back motion. This is however, merely an optical illusion. This technique is most commonly used in the manipulation of a Tendino-Muscle Channel.

CIRCULAR THUMB PRESSURE

In this technique the thumb is used as the manipulating instrument while the body part that is being treated is supported in the palm of the working hand. It is essential to note that the body part is *supported* by the palm of the working hand and *not gripped*, or "held on to" by the working hand. The thumb is maintained in direct alignment with the radius of the practitioner's working arm, and it is not allowed to abduct or adduct unnaturally. This maintains a proper direction of force through the arm and into the hand.

The pad of the thumb is used, or the arch of the thumb, or

the thumb in combination with the thenar eminence of the palm. The size of the area being manipulated will determine the area of the thumb that is used. *Minimal tension* should be experienced in the working hand and arm. This technique is used in the manipulation of specific points on the body; the manipulation of channels on smaller parts of the body, e.g., arms, forearms, hands, feet, shins; and for occasional use on the Bladder Channel on the posterior aspect of the body.

CIRCULAR DIGITAL PRESSURE

In this technique the pads of the three central digits are used to manipulate the area being treated. However, depending on the size of the area being treated you may use as much as the entire palmar aspect of the three central digits, up to and including the metacarpophalangeal joint area of the palm. Although the three digits are used, the major direction of force comes through and from the middle finger. The index and ring fingers are used as secondary or supporting digits rather than initiating digits, and are held closely beside the middle finger in a relaxed manner.

In the more advanced techniques, in which specific points are manipulated to produce directed energetic responses in the patient, the pad of the distal phalange of the index or the middle finger is used to provide directed circular pressure to the specific point. In this case the palm is held in contact with the body, with force being directed into the most distal aspect of the pad of the finger. Note that contact is made with the most distal aspect of the pad of the finger and not with the finger tip.

Circular digital pressure is the most commonly used technique in the administration of Amma. It is used on both large and small areas of the body, with modifications in the technique dependent only on the size of the area being treated.

CIRCULAR PALMAR PRESSURE

In this technique the entire hand is used in the manipulation of a body part, from the pads of the fingers to the heel of the palm. The palm is used as the focus of movement *while the fingers remain relaxed and in complete contact with the body.* Pressure is disseminated evenly throughout the hand rather than being applied by the heel of the palm or the distal pads. The thumb is held beside the digits, and not spread apart from the digits of the working hand or wrapped around the body part being manipulated.

This technique is used in the manipulation of large muscle groups such as the latissimus dorsi, the trapezius, gluteus maximus, the hamstrings, the quadriceps, the adductors, and the abductors, and the most lateral aspects of the body.

CIRCULAR ULNAR
PRESSURE

In this technique the ulnar aspect of the hand, the blade, is used to apply force to the area of the body being manipulated. It is most correctly a highly specific usage of the circular palmar pressure technique. As in circular palmar pressure, the entire hand is held in contact with the body part being manipulated; however, the direction of force is into the area of the hand that ranges from just lateral to the pisiform bone to the metacarpophalangeal joint of the fifth digit. Movement of the hand is in small circles. The hand manipulates the area with which it is directly in contact. It is then lifted and moved to an area one to two inches adjacent to it on a predetermined line of movement. It is most frequently used in the area surrounding the scapulae to release the deeper muscles.

It is significant to note that in the execution of circular digital pressure, circular palmar pressure, and circular ulnar pressure the entire hand is held in contact with the body part being manipulated. *The direction of force and energy into a specific area of the hand is what differentiates each of these techniques.* This is a subtlety that must be developed by the novice practitioner until it becomes "instinctive," that is to say, a natural part of the practice of the manipulation. These techniques are the most frequently used in the adminstration of Amma, and their execution must become highly evolved in the successful practitioner.

CIRCULAR PALM-HEEL
PRESSURE

In this technique the palm-heel is used. Pressure is applied to the body part through the palm-heel, which is directed to making small circles in that area. The hand is lifted and moved to an area one to two inches adjacent to it on a predetermined line of movement. This is frequently used in the release of larger muscle groups, for example, the release of the erector spinae by the practitioner as he or she stands at the head of the prone patient while applying pressure just superior to the posterior superior iliac spine (PSIS), or for the release of the gluteal muscles as the practitioner stands at the patient's side while applying pressure at the base of the buttock into the ischial tuberosity with force being directed toward the PSIS.

Direct Pressure

In this technique, direct contact is made between the part of the hand being used and the body part being manipulated. Direct pressure is issued into the hand, and through it, into the body. The amount of pressure varies with the area of the body being manipulated, and the patient's needs and sensitivities. This is an advanced technique that is used in the direct stimulation of points on the superficial pathways of channels within the energetic system, and in the release of muscle spasm. It is generally followed by circular pressure on the point being held.

This technique should not be used by the novice practitioner. Applied incorrectly, that is, with too much force or with force applied in the wrong direction, it can easily cause damage to the viscera, blood vessels, or nerves. Sufficient information is needed about the effects of pressure on points on the body and the potential results of such pressure. Points that affect Connecting Channels, Tendino-Muscle Channels, or Extraordinary Channels can be stimulated unknowingly, and change body energy. As in all things relating to the contact and treatment of the human body, Amma requires knowledge and caution when being practiced.

DIRECT THUMB PRESSURE/
DIRECT DIGITAL PRESSURE

The administration of this technique employs the use of parts of the distal aspect of the pad of the thumb, index finger, middle finger, or pinky. This technique is typically used for the stimulation of specific points on the superficial branches of the energy channels, and, depending on the area of the body being manipulated, either the whole pad, the most distal aspect of the pad, or a portion of the most distal aspect of the pad may be used. This is entirely dependent upon the location of the point being treated. For example, the stimulation of a point located at the inner canthus of the eye would require the use of *a portion* of the most distal aspect of the pad of the pinky because of the small size of the body being treated. However, the pad of the thumb or middle finger could be used to stimulate a point located on the inner thigh, arm, chest, or back. The appropriate administration of this technique requires great strength and control in the completely relaxed hand.

Stroking

The stroking techniques involve passing the hand or part of the hand over an area of the body. The force issued into the hand is distributed equally throughout the hand or part of the hand being used so that pressure remains constant and even throughout the hand. For example, if the entire hand is used, the pressure that the patient feels coming from the palm of the hand will be equal to the amount of pressure that he feels coming from the palmar aspect of the fingers.

THUMB STROKING

Thumb stroking involves the use of the entire palmar aspect of the thumb: the pad, the arch, and the proximal phalange. Pressure that is issued into the thumb is distributed equally throughout the thumb. This technique is most commonly used in the treatment of the muscles of the forehead, the face, and the medial aspect of the foot. Without the application of deep pressure, this technique can be used freely during the course of the treatment.

DIGITAL STROKING

This technique employs the use of the palmar aspect of the three phalanges of the second, third, fourth, and fifth digits or the two most distal phalanges of these same digits. A sweeping motion covering a large surface area may be used, or an up-and-back motion may be used. There is a light contact, with little or no pressure, between the working hand and the body part being manipulated. This is frequently used in the reduction of edema in the extremities. In this case, the direction of movement is with the venous flow, that is, toward the trunk of the body, in order to facilitate lymphatic drainage.

FULL PALMAR STROKING

Palmar stroking involves the use of the entire palmar aspect of the hand *in full contact* with the body. A gentle gliding motion is used over the surface of the area being manipulated. In the correct administration of this technique, a "molding effect" takes place in which the hand molds to the configuration of the area of the body as it passes over it. This is resultant of maintaining a completely relaxed hand. This is a highly relaxing technique often employed on the posterior surface of the body in long sweeping motions.

LOOSE FIST STROKING

The novice practitioner may find that his fingers tire easily during the course of a treatment. If this is the case, he may alternate techniques being used with loose fist stroking, particularly on areas of large muscle development such as the thighs, back, and buttocks.

A very relaxed fist is formed, sufficiently relaxed that no tension is experienced in the forearm. The fingers of the hand are flexed toward the palm, without flexing the metacarpophalangeal joint area of the hand. There is a straight line, therefore, between the wrist and the proximal head of the second phalange of each of the four digits. The thumb is held in a relaxed fashion beside the index finger. The area of contact is the middle phalange of the second, third, and fourth digits. The key here lies in maintaining the hand position with an inner strength that moves through the body and arm, into the proximal head of the second phalanges of the fingers.

Use either a short up-and-back motion or the spiraling movement of circular pressure, keeping constant contact between the working area of the hand and the body part being manipulated.

Embracing

In this technique the hand is molded to the contours of the body, and a drawing, or suction, motion is applied with the palm of the hand, drawing the body part up into the palm. This technique is a palmar technique: no finger tip pressure is applied. To administer this technique successfully, it is essential that the fingers are completely relaxed.

PALMAR EMBRACE   In this technique the thenar and the hypothenar areas of the hand are used in opposition to one another in a drawing motion that produces a "vertical" suction effect. The focus of movement is solely in the palm of the hand with some contact being made by the proximal phalange of the second, third, fourth, and fifth digits. The fingers of the hand must be held relaxed in the administration of this technique to insure that no fingertip pressure is applied.

This technique is effectively used in the release and relaxation of small muscle groups such as the brachialis in the forearm, or the calves in smaller women and children.

THENAR EMBRACE   This technique produces a horizontal drawing motion rather than the vertical drawing motion that is produced in the palmar embrace. In this technique the thenar area and the palm-heel oppose the metacarpophalangeal joint area of the palm and the most proximal phalange of the second, third, fourth, and fifth digits to produce a drawing motion. This is effectively used in the release and relaxation of larger muscle groups—the upper trapezius, calves on larger women and men, or the posterior aspect of the arms.

Percussion

In these techniques a light tapping motion is applied to the surface of the body, sending a vibration through the body to produce a stimulating effect. The novice practitioner should practice these techniques on his own body before using them on his patients. Practice will insure that the techniques produce the vibratory effect without the sharp pain that may accompany an incorrectly applied technique.

CUPPING   In this technique the hand is held in a relaxed "pyramid" form. The four digits are held together with the fingers extended. The thumb is held beside the index finger. A slight bend is held at the metacarpophalangeal joint, forming an angle of approximately one hundred and thirty-five degrees. Viewed laterally a modified "A" shape will be seen. A hollow is created at the center of the palm. When this technique is executed properly, the palm *never* contacts the body. This is applied in a *continuous rhythmic* manner, with the two hands alternately striking the body. As a result it produces a highly stimulating yet relaxing effect when used properly.

This technique can be used on the back, buttocks, thighs, legs, and shoulders. In addition, when it is applied to the posterior aspect of the thorax, it is used effectively to stimulate release of mucus and mucopurulent material from the lungs.

CHOPPING   The blade, or ulnar aspect, of the hand is used in this technique. The wrist is held in a relaxed manner, allowing the hand free movement at the joint. The fingers, while held together, are relaxed. The striking area extends from the area just lateral to the pisiform bone to the distal aspect of the fifth digit. Two hands strike in an alternating fashion in a continuous and rhythmic manner. This produces a stimulating yet relaxing effect when administered properly. Like cupping, this technique can be used on the back, buttocks, thighs, calves, and shoulders. However, neither cupping nor chopping should be used directly over the spine itself.

CHAPTER NINE
Principles of Treatment

1. A novice practitioner of any form of manipulative therapy who thinks of the treatment of the human body most often thinks of using the hands, arms, and shoulders. However, hands-on manipulation involves the interaction of two human beings. It is not simply the manipulation of one human being by the hands and arms of another. The entire body of the practitioner is involved; the entire energy system of the practitioner is involved. It is necessary, therefore, that a high degree of personal health be maintained.

It is not uncommon for the practitioner to suffer from congestion in and problems with the genitourinary area *as a result* of allowing his own health and energy to fall well below optimum levels. For this reason, the primary and overriding principle to be held by the practitioner is the maintenance of optimum levels of physical, emotional, and energetic health.

2. The hand works as a tool. The guiding force of movement is the body, the torso, the the *tan tien*.[1] The hand itself does not initiate movement; neither does the arm or the shoulder.

3. Proper postural alignment must be maintained. The shoulders should be held back and down, the rib cage dropped, and the abdomen, perineum, and anus open and relaxed. This draws the center of gravity into the lower torso where it should be maintained. Weight should be evenly distributed between the feet.

4. The hand remains relaxed and in contact with the body as much as possible. This applies in stroking, pressure, and embracing techniques. A "molding effect" takes place as a result of having a completely relaxed hand. Note the differentiation between a completely relaxed hand and a limp hand. A

hand that is completely relaxed is one that is controlled with minimal muscular tension. In the limp hand there is no control. The relaxed hand should be maintained throughout the treatment.

5. The palm should be held in contact with the body as much as possible, wherever possible, regardless of the portion of the hand being used in the manipulation.

6. The hand should be used to palpate as well as to treat. At all times during the treatment, full attention should be placed in the hand to feel the body for swellings, temperature changes, and skin quality differences. As a result, the hand becomes a primary information-gathering device.

7. Both hands should always be in contact with the patient; while one hand works, the other should be maintaining light contact with the limb or body part being manipulated. Differentiate between gripping the body part or holding onto the patient, and maintaining light contact.

8. Techniques should be applied rhythmically, both within the application of any given technique and in the transition from one technique to another.

9. Treatment patterns should be in the general direction of the muscle fibers rather than across the fibers or in opposition to the direction of the muscle fibers.

10. Understand what you wish to accomplish through the use of a technique before using it. For example, be fully aware that your treatment technique is aimed at the relaxation of a muscle or movement of the energy in a specific direction.

Endnote   [1] *Tan tien* is considered the "Golden Cauldron" in Chinese meditative practice. It is the center of energy, balance, and gravity in the human body, and is utilized in all instinctive, moving, and sexual activities. It has been mistakenly called a "point" located two inches below the navel. However, it is more correctly considered a repository of energy encompassing the entire area, three-dimensionally, below the navel to the floor of the torso and is inclusive of the lower abdomen, the genitals, and the buttocks.

CHAPTER TEN
The Basic Amma

IN the administration of the Basic Amma, the practitioner treats in both a seated and a standing position. Whether seated or standing, proper postural alignment must be maintained. The shoulders and scapulae should be held back and down, the rib cage dropped, and the abdomen, perineum, buttocks, and anus relaxed. In the seated position the feet should be placed comfortably on the floor without crossing the legs or ankles. In a standing position weight should be evenly distributed between the feet, knees slightly bent. The head should be held erect, and the hands, arms, and shoulders relaxed.

The treatment begins with the patient lying comfortably in the supine position. He should be dressed in loose, comfortable clothing. The practitioner is seated behind the patient's head.

1. Treatment begins with the patient's head in a central position. Place the hands on the patient's head with the pads of the thumbs in contact with the midpoint between the eyebrows. The radial edges of the thumb nails, the radial edges of the thumbs, and the thenar eminences are touching. The thumbs are in line with the midsagittal plane on the forehead. The palms are resting on the forehead, with the fingers resting on the lateral aspects of the face.

Using thumb stroking with the pads of the thumbs, gently stroke over the eyebrows, starting at this center point and moving toward the temples and into the lateral hairline. Repeat this movement five times.

The stroke moves horizontally across the forehead, and into the lateral hairline. There is a tendency for the horizontal stroking across the forehead to lead into a *caudal* stroke into the hairline moving toward the ears. Care should be taken to avoid this.

Step 1

1-1

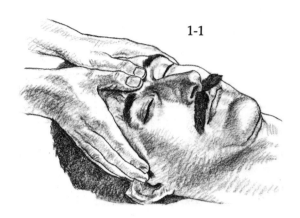

1-2

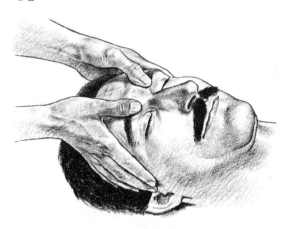

1-3

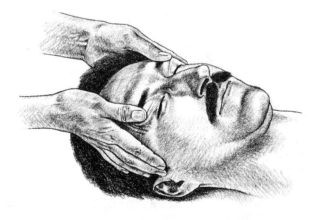

1-4

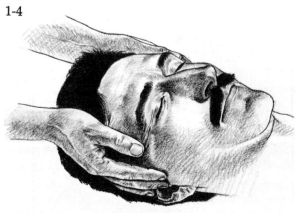

2. Place the hands in the initial position described in Step 1. Hyperextend the thumbs at the distal phalange and stroke *above* the eyebrows, in the superciliary arch, moving from the midsagittal line to the lateral hairline. Repeat five times.

The *placement of pressure* from the pads of the thumbs to the arch of the thumbs permits stroking of the area just above the eyebrow rather than on the eyebrow, thus differentiating the stroke used in Step 1 from the stroke used in Step 2.

Step 2

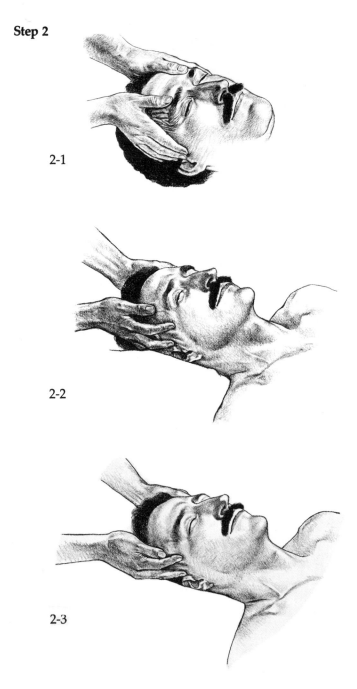

2-1

2-2

2-3

Step 3

3. Place the hands in the initial position described in Step 1. Beginning at the midpoint between the eyebrows and using thumb stroking with the pads of the thumbs, stroke up the midsagittal line of the forehead approximately one inch, and then stroke across the forehead into the lateral hairline. Repeat this movement, moving up the forehead in one-half inch intervals until the superior hairline (the hairline at the top of the head) is reached. End this group of strokes with thumb stroking at the level of the superior hairline. Repeat five times.

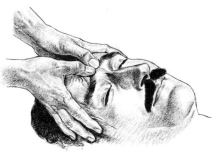

3-1

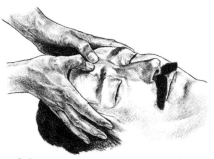

3-2

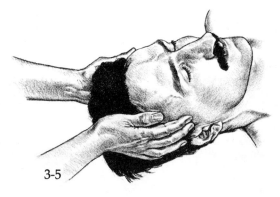

3-5

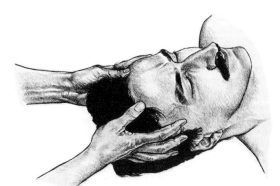

3-3

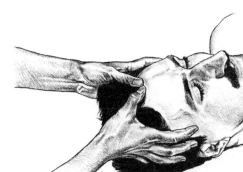

3-6

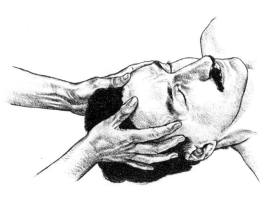

3-4

3-7

4. Begin with pads of the distal phalanges of the three central digits on a line just above the eyebrows. Using circular digital pressure, move toward the superior hairline in half-inch intervals. One hand works while the other hand is used to support the lateral aspect of the patient's face and head on the side opposite to the side being worked. Repeat the manipulation of each side of the forehead five times.

Remember that the circles are intended to move the soft tissue underlying the epidermis of the forehead. Once the digits have been placed, a circling motion is made, moving the skin and the muscle underlying the fingers. After circling five or six times, the hand is moved approximately one-half inch and another series of circles is made. This results in a *palpation* of the area under treatment as well as the administration of a hand technique. The underlying skeletal structure is touched and its surface changes noted.

Step 4

4-1
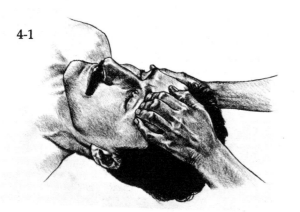

4-2
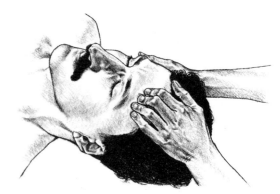

4-3
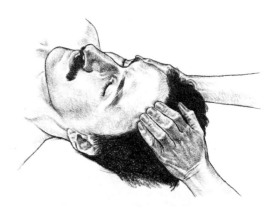

5. Place the hands in the position described in Step 1. Using the thumb stroking technique, working with one thumb at a time, alternating working hands, stroke up the midsagittal line to the superior hairline. As soon as the thumb of one hand reaches the hairline, the other thumb begins its vertical stroke. The fingers of both rest on the patient's head as much as possible. Repeat five times.

Step 5

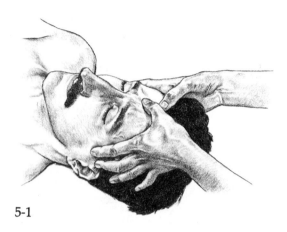

5-1

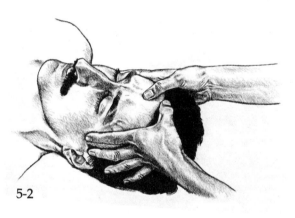

5-2

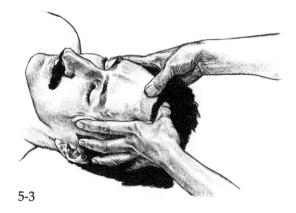

5-3

6. Place the thumbs on the midsagittal line of the forehead *at the superior hairline*. Hands are resting on the head. Using the thumb stroking technique, stroke laterally from the midpoint of the forehead at the superior hairline to the lateral hairline. Both hands work simultaneously. Care should be taken to avoid stroking caudally (toward the ears). Repeat five times.

The manipulation of the forehead has the primary effect of relaxing the temporalis and the frontalis portion of the epicranius muscle, which promotes relaxation of both the galea aponeurotica and the occipital muscle at the base of the occiput.

In addition to the muscular relaxation, these techniques help drain the frontal sinus cavities, providing relief for those who suffer with sinus headache or congestion. This should be an area of concentration on patients who suffer with headache centered at the forehead or the back of the head or neck, eyestrain, and sinus congestion due to allergies or common cold. Tension in the frontalis muscle is generally reflective of generalized muscular tension. Therefore, manipulation of this area soothes and relaxes the local area as well as the remainder of the body.

Step 6

6-1

6-2

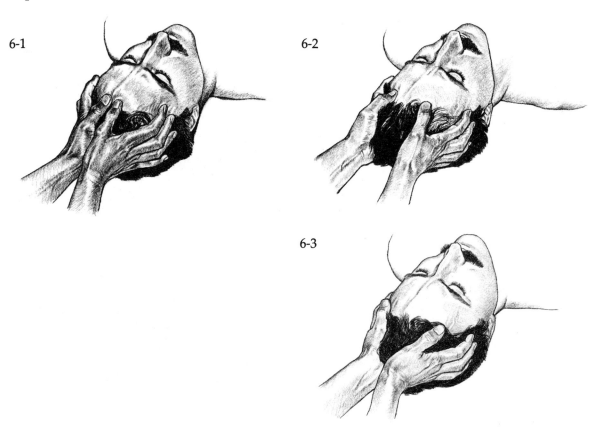

6-3

7. Place the pads of the three central digits at the temples with the index finger in line with the outer canthus of the eye and the third finger just superior to the tragus of the ear. You will feel a slight indentation just above the zygomatic process of the temporal bone. Using circular digital pressure, manipulate the temple area from the level of the eye to the superior hairline, moving in half-inch intervals. One hand works while the other remains in light contact with the lateral aspect of the face and head. Repeat the manipulation of each temple five times.

Manipulation in this area has the primary effect of relaxing the temporalis muscle. This has been found to have profound effects in overall relaxation. Simply holding the temple area for fifteen to forty-five seconds produces a calming effect on the entire body. Manipulation here should be emphasized in the treatment of patients suffering with headache in the temporal region, bruxism, and temporomandibular joint syndrome, as well as for those who are experiencing emotional tension.

Step 7

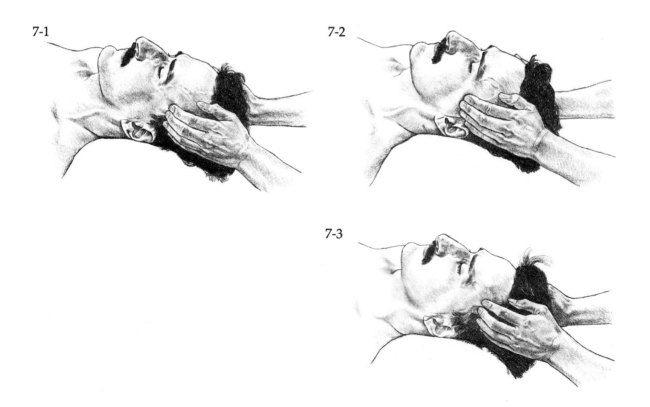

7-1

7-2

7-3

8. Turn the head to one side, making sure that the head is not overturned and that the patient is comfortable at all times. In turning, support the patient's head by cupping the ears with both hands. Avoid applying pressure to the ears by cupping your hands before placing them over the ears. There is frequently a tendency to turn the patient's head almost to a point of traction. This is unnecessary and causes undue discomfort for the patient. In addition, it produces tension in the soft tissues of the lateral aspect of the neck that makes manipulation of the sternocleidomastoid muscle more difficult.

Using circular digital pressure, manipulate the area at the posterior border of the sternocleidomastoid muscle from the base of the occiput to the area just above the clavicle. Repeat the manipulation of one side of the neck five times before turning the patient's head to treat the other side of the neck.

Maintaining palmar contact in this area is difficult, depending on the size of the patient being treated. It may be necessary to begin with the distal aspects of the digits, perhaps the distal and middle phalanges, and extend the contact to include the proximal phalange and metacarpophalangeal joint area of the hand as the movement proceeds toward the clavicle.

The manipulation of this area has multiple effects and purpose. Through the manipulation, tension in the sternocleidomastoid muscle and the platysma is relieved. This will relax the neck, upper chest, jaw, chin, and throat. All of these areas tend to be centers of tension in many people. For those suffering with shoulder tension, neck tension, and bruxism, this is a particularly effective technique. Manipulation here also promotes the drainage of the cervical lymph nodes, which may become swollen secondary to allergy or upper respiratory congestion and/or infection.

Step 8

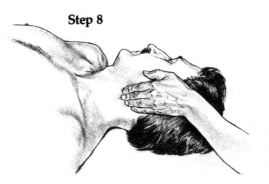

8-1

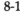

8-2

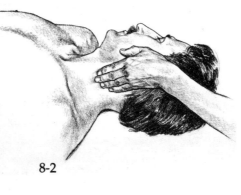

8-3

9. Beginning at the temples, treat the area around the ear, using circular digital pressure on a line that approximates the path of the squamosal suture. Careful palpation of the area will demonstrate a slight sulcus at the suture line. The middle finger of your working hand remains in contact with the suture line. Work around the ear and down to the base of the occiput. Continue by manipulating the base of the occiput toward the center of the back of the neck with the fingertips. Repeat five times. Work only one side at a time, supporting the patient's head with the hand that is not working.

This technique works a portion of the superficial aspect of the Gall Bladder Channel. The Gall Bladder Channel reflects and affects emotional energy. Manipulation here produces emotional and physical calm.

The manipulation at the base of the occiput releases the splenius capitis muscle, the origin of the upper trapezius muscle and the smaller deep muscles that connect the skull to the cervical vertebrae (longissimus capitis, spinalis capitis, semispinalis capitis, rectus capitis posterior major and minor, obliquus capitis superior). The combined effect is one of total release of the base of the skull at the level of the occiput with muscular relaxation extending down toward the lower aspects of the thorax.

Manipulation of this area should be used with patients suffering with emotional stress, headache, chronic or acute shoulder tension, back tension, or impingement of the cervical nerves, and for those suffering with Bladder-related dysfunction—infections, menstrual problems, and prostatic disorders.

Step 9

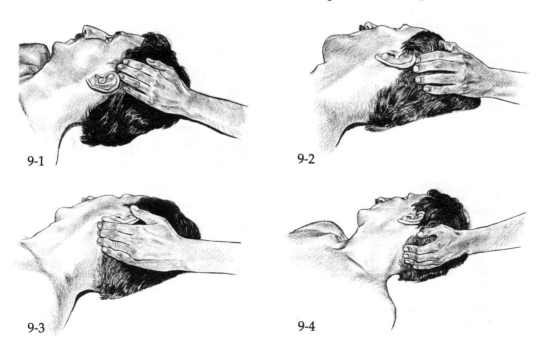

9-1

9-2

9-3

9-4

Step 10

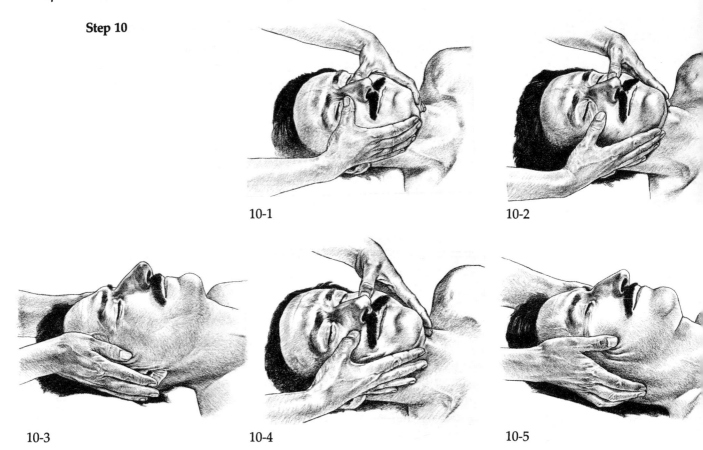

10-1

10-2

10-3

10-4

10-5

10. Using the thumb stroking technique, stroke laterally over the nose and cheekbones toward the temples. Begin with the pad of each thumb in contact with the nasal bones, with the thumbs molding to the contours of the maxilla and zygomatic bones. It will be necessary to hyperextend the thumbs in order to mold to the contours of the face. Stroke laterally, following the contours of the bony structure of the cheeks. End the stroke in the hairline at the temples. Two stroke patterns are used: one follows the superior aspect of the maxilla and zygomatic bones, and one adheres to the distal aspect of the zygomatic arch. Repeat each stroke five times.

Manipulation here affects the nasal sinuses, reducing swelling and facilitating the drainage of mucus. This should be an area of focus for those suffering with chronic or acute rhinitis. It is highly beneficial to people suffering with sinus headache. In addition, manipulation in this area relaxes the small facial muscles. The face is a center of tension, and manipulation promotes relaxation in general.

11. Beginning with the left hand and using circular digital pressure, employing as much of the palmar aspect of the three central digits as possible, manipulate the sternal area. Movement proceeds downward, from the interclavicular notch to the xyphoid process.

The left and right hands alternate in the manipulation down the sternum. Repeat three times, alternating hands.

Step 11

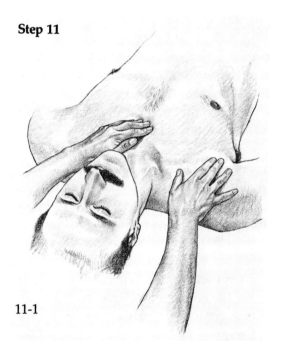

11-1

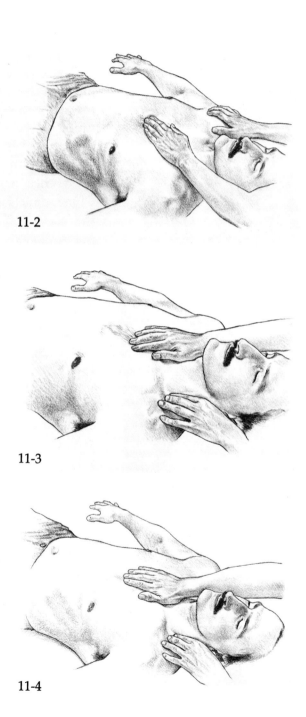

11-2

11-3

11-4

12. Using circular digital pressure, treat the upper chest from the sternum to the shoulders, working in the intercostal spaces. Work one side at a time, using the right hand to manipulate the patient's right side, and the left hand to manipulate the patient's left side. Manipulation is in the intercostal spaces between the first and second, second and third, and third and fourth ribs. Repeat the treatment of each space two or three times. Alternate right and left sides as you move from the clavicular area to the lower aspects of the chest to encourage muscular balance throughout the course of the manipulation.

It is difficult to use this technique in the manner described on large-breasted women because of the difficulty in contacting the bony structure of the thorax. In this case, move down the thorax only as far as you can without manipulating over the breast tissue. In some women, this may mean that only the first-second and second-third intercostal spaces may be accessible to manipulation.

The chest tends to be a center of tension. In both the classical Chinese and Hindu systems of thought, it is considered to be the center of emotional energy within the physical body. Manipulation of this area will disperse emotional tension that is held in the chest. There is a strong emotional component in illness and disease, and since physical manipulation will release much pent-up energy contained within this area, it should be repeated during the course of the treatment.

All of the Arm Yin Tendino-Muscle Channels enter into the upper chest: the Lung Channel, the Heart Channel, and the Heart Envelope Channel. Therefore, manipulation of the sternum and chest is used clinically in the treatment of respiratory problems; coughs due to colds, allergies, asthma, pneumonia, cardiovascular problems; and high or low blood pressure and poor circulation. Treatment here is useful when dealing with gastrointestinal disorders such as sluggish digestion, irritable bowel syndrome, colitis, and constipation.

Frequently a patient will be unable to specify the nature of a physical ailment but still feels *unwell*. In this case, manipulation of this, as well as other areas involved in the release of emotional stress, should be treated with particular attention.

The practitioner moves to a standing position at the patient's right side.

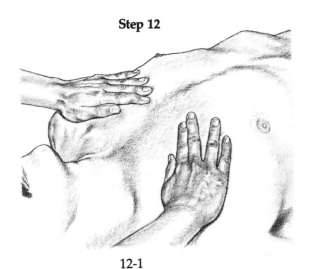

Step 12

12-1

13. Support the patient's right hand, palm upturned, in the palm of your right hand without grasping it tightly with your fingers. Working with the left hand, and beginning in the area of the deltopectoral groove, work up to the level of the middle deltoid, and then down the anterolateral aspect of the arm to the thenar eminence at the thumb. Use circular thumb pressure with the left thumb or circular digital pressure with the digits of the left hand. Repeat the manipulation of this pathway five times.

This follows aspects of the Superficial and Tendino-Muscle Pathways of the Lung Channel which fall within the large muscles of the radial aspect of the arm and forearm. Manipulation of this area benefits those who suffer with respiratory difficulties, including coughs due to colds or smoking as well as pulmonary pathologic conditions. For people who live in densely populated areas where air pollution tends to be high, or for people who smoke, manipulation of this area will help to strengthen the lungs.

Step 13

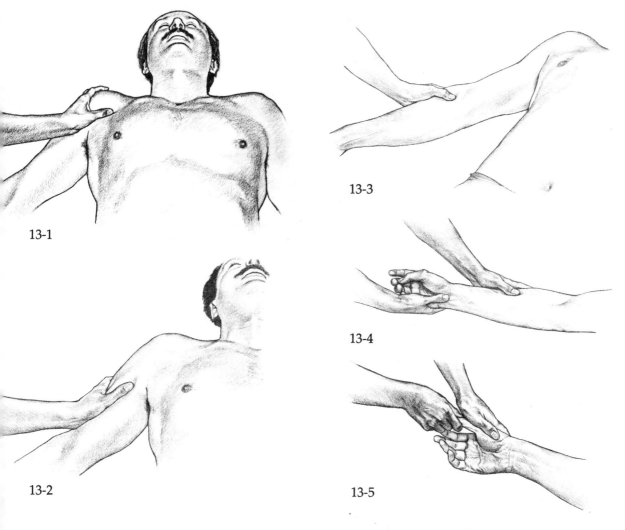

13-1

13-2

13-3

13-4

13-5

14. Support the patient's upturned right hand in the palm of your left hand without grasping it tightly. Using circular palmar pressure, and beginning with the fingertips of the right hand at the axilla, treat the medial (ulnar) portion of the anterior arm down to the little finger. Repeat five times.

The manipulation follows the Superficial and Tendino-Muscle Pathways of the Heart Channel. This will both relax and strengthen the heart. It is used for patients suffering with cardiovascular problems, and for those who experience anxiety or depression.

Step 14

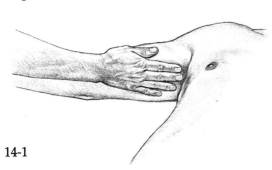

14-1

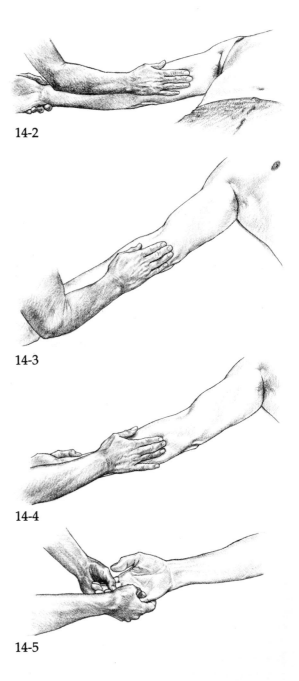

14-2

14-3

14-4

14-5

15. Support the patient's hand at the wrist with two hands. Turn the palmar surface down and flex the wrist slightly. Hold the patient's hand and forearm off the table while allowing the elbow to rest on the table. Using circular thumb pressure with the distal aspects of the pads of the thumbs, manipulate in the spaces between the carpal bones in the wrist joint.

Manipulation between the carpal bones promotes the circulation of blood and energy in the extremity, frequently resulting in an increase of peripheral body temperature. Therefore, this is beneficial for those suffering with poor circulation in the hands and fingers.

Step 15

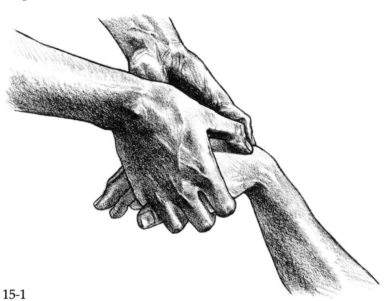

15-1

16. Using circular thumb pressure with the distal aspects of the pads of the thumbs, manipulate in between the metacarpal bones of the hand, moving from the carpal bones to the metacarpophalangeal joint area on the dorsum of the hand. Treat each space two or three times.

Step 16

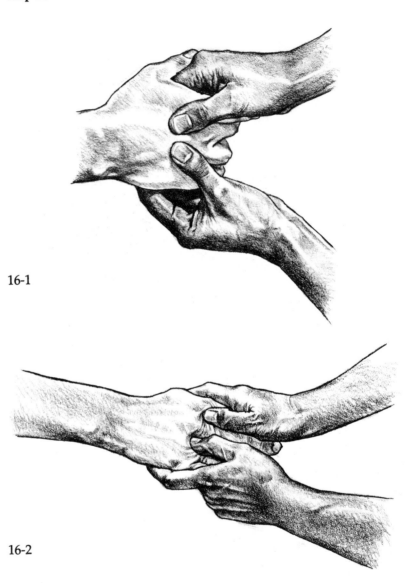

16-1

16-2

17. Treatment of the hand ends with a general manipulation of each finger on the anterior and posterior surfaces as well as the medial and lateral surfaces. Repeat each finger two or three times. The fingers are treated in the following order to promote musculo-skeletal balance: middle finger, ring finger, index finger, little finger, thumb.

Energy passes from Yin to Yang and Yang to Yin in the fingers and toes. Manipulation of the digits is considered to be important because it frees the energy and stimulates circulation of blood and other body fluids. Manipulation relaxes the musculature and reduces swelling in the joints. Treatment here is important for those who suffer with arthritis in the hands.

Step 17

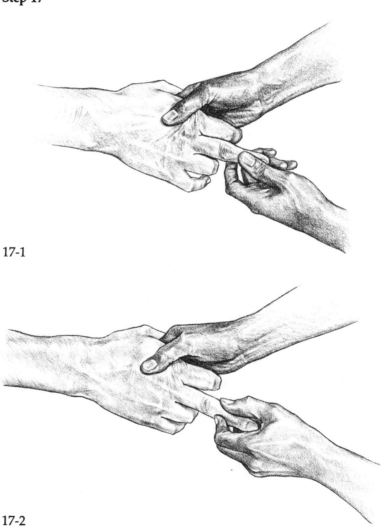

17-1

17-2

18. Using circular palmar pressure with the right hand, manipulate the chest and abdomen. Begin at the sternum and proceed down the center line of the body to the pubic bone. It is essential that a gentle stroke be used, because of the delicate nature of the soft tissues of the abdomen. Repeat this pathway five times.

Step 18

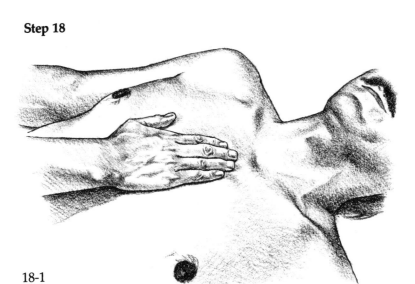

18-1

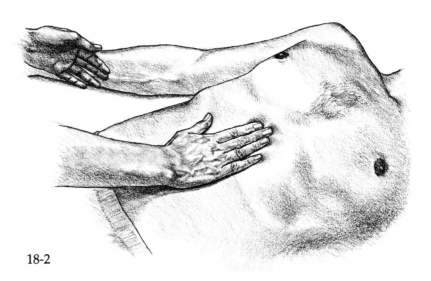

18-2

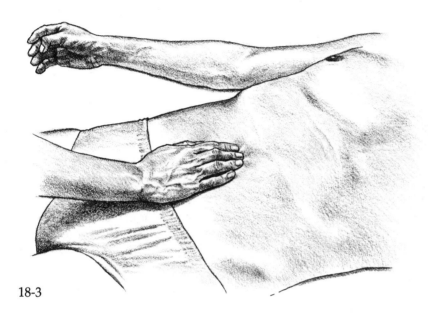

18-3

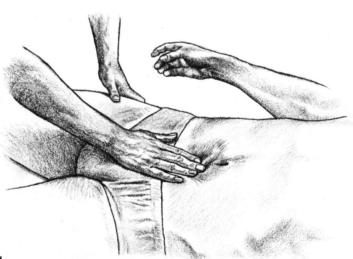

18-4

19. Place both hands on the abdomen with the fingertips distal to the lower ribs. Palms are held in full contact with the abdomen at all times. Using palmar embrace, manipulate the abdomen, creating a wavelike motion with your hands.

You must envision the movement of the contents of the colon through the ascending colon, to the transverse colon, to the descending colon. Both hands work in alternation, with the left hand moving the contents up and medially, and the right hand moving the contents medially and downward. The result is a kneading movement that resembles the kneading movements manifested by cats.

The intention here is to stimulate movement of the contents of the colon in order to facilitate the release of feces and flatus. Patients should be reminded to try to relax when the abdomen is treated. They may feel the desire to lock the anus to prevent the release of gas. They may feel embarrassed and try to prevent this natural occurrence. This behavior, however, accomplishes just the opposite of what the Amma practitioner is trying to do. The practitioner should remind the patient that the release of flatus is a natural and *desirable* result of this portion of the treatment. They should try to allow it to take place if it must. *It is in this kind of situation that the practitioner must utilize his most professional demeanor.*

The abdomen is often a very sensitive area, and a gentle

Step 19

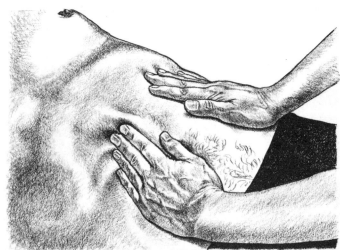

19-1

stroke should be used. However, the depth of manipulation can be geared to the needs of the patient. As the area is manipulated, the patient relaxes, then the depth of massage will increase.

Occasionally you will find a patient who experiences a particular sensitivity in one area of the abdomen when it is manipulated. By and large, any sensitivity should dissipate as the manipulation proceeds. If it does not, continue with the remainder of the treatment, and refer the patient to a physician for a physical examination.

Manipulation that follows the direction of the colon will stimulate peristaltic activity. This is beneficial for all patients, since dietary deficiencies and stress-related difficulties are prevalent in today's society and are frequently the cause of constipation or sluggish bowels with insufficient fecal elimination. This technique can be used with patients suffering with irritable bowel syndrome, chronic constipation, ulcer, colitis, flatulence, and hemorrhoids.

For those people suffering with diarrhea, the direction of the manipulation should be reversed—that is, upward and medially on the left side of the abdomen, and medially and downward on the right. This produces the effect whereby the contents of the colon are retained, thereby increasing fluid reabsorbtion from fecal matter within the colon.

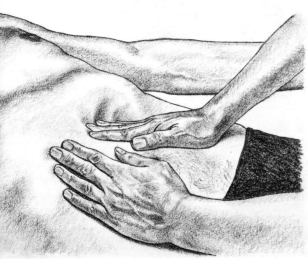

19-2

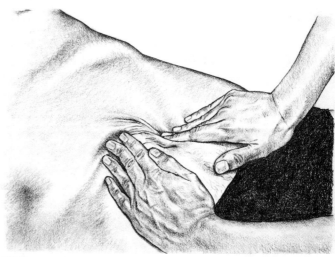

19-3

20. Manipulate the antero-lateral aspect of the right thigh from the hip to the knee, using circular palmar pressure with the left hand. Begin with the fingers of the left hand at the level of the anterior superior iliac spine (ASIS). Support the inner thigh or the lower leg with the right hand. Repeat five times.

Manipulation in this area relaxes the large muscles of the antero-lateral thigh. This includes portions of the sartorius, rectus femoris, vastus intermedius, and vastus lateralis. Circulation to the lower limb is increased, and lymphatic drainage is stimulated. Manipulation of this area is useful for those suffering with pain or dysfunction of the hips and knees.

The Tendino-Muscle and Superficial aspects of the Stomach Channel are affected through the manipulation of this portion of the thigh, and will therefore benefit patients who suffer with gastrointestinal disturbances.

Step 20

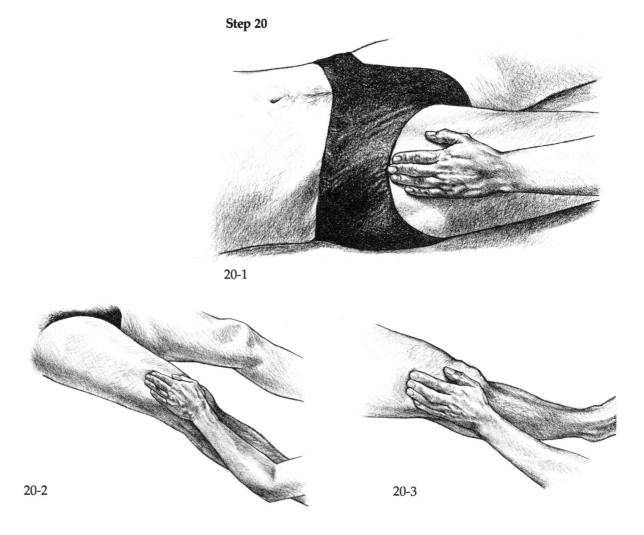

20-1

20-2

20-3

21. Support the lateral aspect of the thigh with the left hand. Using circular palmar pressure with the right hand, manipulate the medial aspect of the thigh from the groin to the inner knee. This area tends to be sensitive in many people, and care should be taken to avoid deep or excessive manipulation. Repeat five times.

Manipulation here affects portions of the adductor longus and adductor magnus, the gracilis, and the distal portion of the sartorius. Treatment in this area facilitates the drainage of lymphatic fluid through the inguinal lymph nodes. This is useful for patients suffering with systemic infection, genitourinary tract infections, and problems related to the lower limbs.

The Tendino-Muscle and Superficial aspects of the Liver and Spleen Channels are affected in the manipulation of this area of the body.

Directed manipulation of the area just distal to the groin and the area just proximal to the medial epicondyle on the femur promotes circulation of these energies, helping those suffering with a broad range of genitourinary tract difficulties.

Step 21

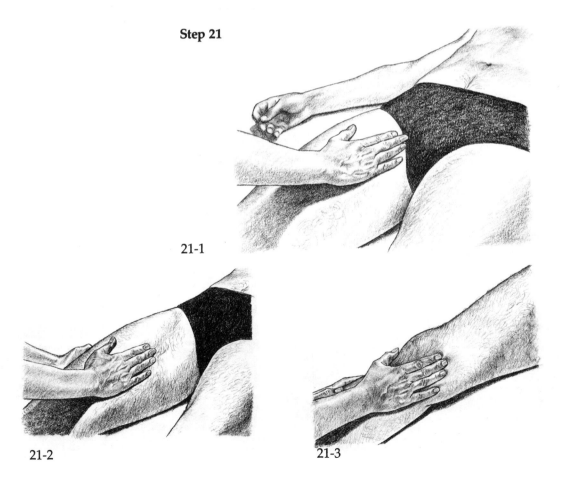

21-1

21-2

21-3

22. Using circular palmar pressure with the left hand, manipulate the lateral aspect of the hip and thigh down to the knee. Begin lateral to the anterior superior iliac spine (ASIS), on the coronal plane of the body. Support the inner leg with the right hand. Repeat five times.

Manipulation of this area relaxes the tensor fascia latae, the ilio-tibial tract, and the vastus lateralis. Manipulation of this area is essential in the treatment of both knee and hip dysfunction.

Portions of the Tendino-Muscle and Superficial aspects of the Gall Bladder Channel lie in this area. This channel tends to most clearly reflect and affect the emotional aspect of an individual. Manipulation of this area of the body will frequently have a soothing effect on the patient, reducing emotional stress.

Step 22

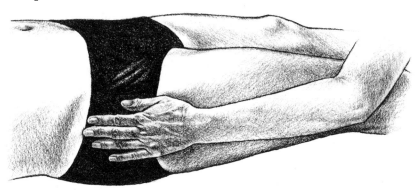

22-1

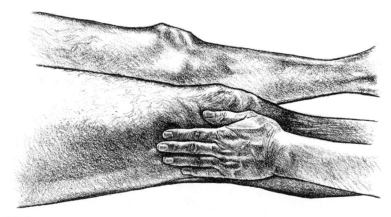

22-2

23. Support the inner leg with the right hand. Beginning with the left hand at the ASIS and using circular palmar pressure, follow the course of the sartorius muscle down to its insertion at the medial aspect of the tibia. The hand begins at the hip on the *antero-lateral* aspect of the body with the fingers facing in an upward direction. However, manipulation of this muscle ends at the *inner* knee with the fingers facing downward. As the hand moves down the thigh following the course of the sartorius, it rotates, using the palm-heel as its point of rotation. (*Instructions for this step continue on page 162.*)

Step 23

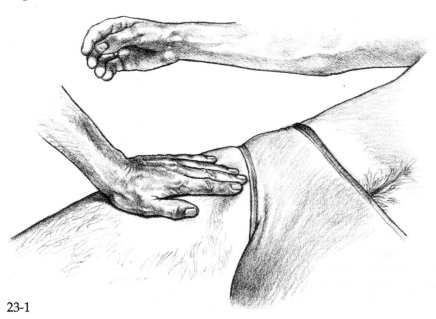

23-1

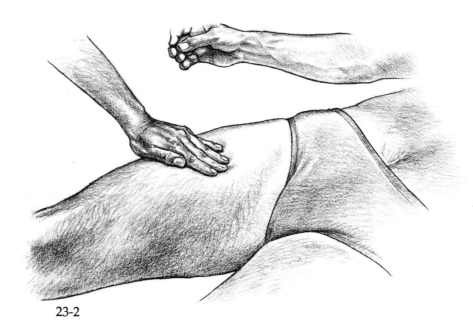

23-2

Rotation begins as the hand reaches the midthigh. Treatment ends just distal to the head of the tibia with the fingertips facing the foot. The palmar surface of the fingers remains in contact with the sartorius at all times.

The sartorius, the longest muscle in the body, crosses two major joints of the lower extremity, the hip and the knee. The manipulation and relaxation of this muscle affects both joints, and is useful in the treatment of any dysfunction involving either one.

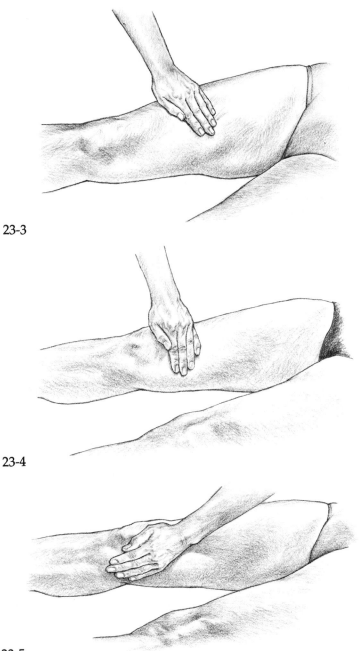

23-3

23-4

23-5

24. Using circular digital pressure with the right hand, manipulate the inner knee, moving from the area superior to the medial epicondyle of the femur, to the area just distal to the head of the tibia. Portions of the tendon insertions of the sartorius, gracilis, semimembranosus, and semitendinosus are manipulated. Repeat five times.

Circular digital pressure should also be directed to the area just medial to the patella. This affects the vastus medialis and the ligamentous tissue overlying the patella.

The manipulation of this area promotes the free flow of synovial fluid surrounding the knee joint. Because of its weight-bearing function, the knee is one of the most highly stressed areas in the body. It is easily injured and is frequently the site in which arthritis develops. Because of the fibrous nature of the tissues which form the joint, healing is slow and difficult. Circulation of the body fluids as a result of the manipulation is extremely important, both therapeutically and preventatively.

Step 24

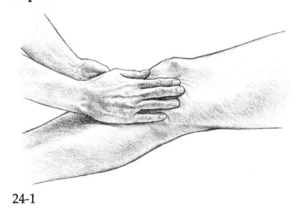

24-1

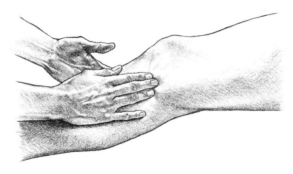

24-2

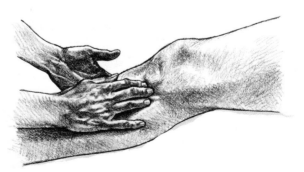

24-3

25. Supporting the inner leg with the right hand, use circular digital pressure with the left hand to manipulate the lateral aspect of the knee joint. In doing so, the vastus lateralis, tensor fascia latae, and portions of the patellar ligament are manipulated.

Step 25

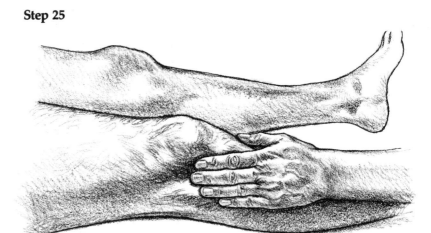

25-1

26. Supporting the leg with the right hand and using circular digital pressure with the left, manipulate the lower leg, beginning at the lateral aspect of the knee and moving toward the lateral malleolus. Repeat five times.

The manipulation of this area follows the tibialis anterior and the extensor digitorum longus. The manipulation of these muscles has a direct effect on the relaxation of the ankle and foot, both of which tend to be highly stressed areas of the body because of their weight-bearing function.

Step 26

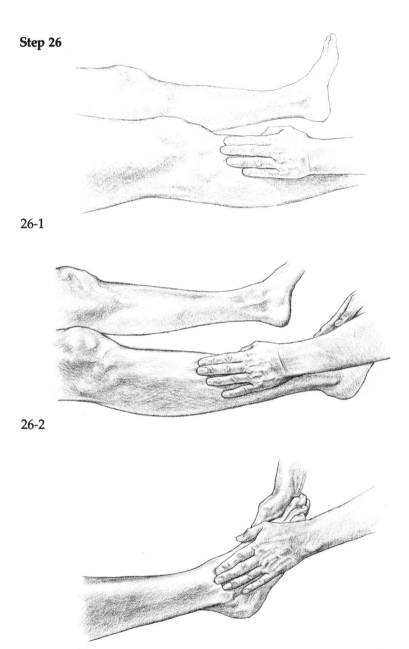

26-1

26-2

26-3

27. Manipulate the medial aspect of the lower leg from the head of the tibia to the medial malleolus, using circular digital pressure with the right hand. Support the leg with the left hand. Repeat five times.

Step 27

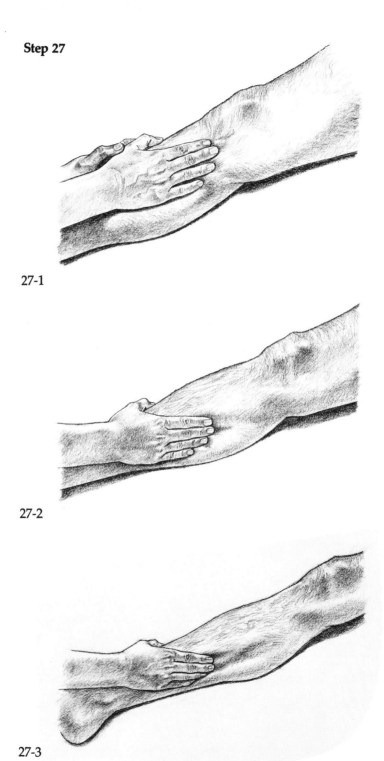

27-1

27-2

27-3

28. Using circular digital pressure with the left hand, manipulate around the lateral malleolus, describing an arc approximately one-half inch distal to it. Begin at the calcaneus, and move caudally toward the toes. Manipulate around the medial malleolus in the same way, using the right hand. Repeat the manipulation of each area five times.

Portions of the Superficial aspect of the Bladder Channel lie on the lateral aspect of the ankle. Portions of the Superficial aspect of the Kidney Channel lie on the medial aspect of the ankle. Manipulation of these areas is used in the treatment of a complete range of genitourinary tract dysfunctions.

Step 28

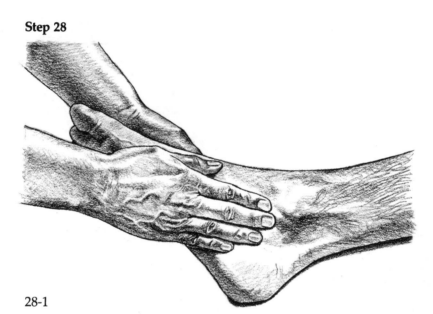

28-1

Move to the end of the table.

29. Support the plantar surface of the foot with the palm of the left hand. Using circular digital pressure with the right hand, manipulate the dorsal surface of the foot from the ankle to the toes. Work between the tarsal bones, and between the metatarsals. Complete the manipulation of the dorsum of the foot with a manipulation of each toe, following the 3-4-2-5-1 pattern used on the fingers (see Step 17).

Portions of the Bladder, Gall Bladder, Stomach, Liver, and Spleen Channels lie on the dorsum of the foot. As with the hands and fingers, manipulation of the feet and toes is significant in the circulation of energy, for it is with the digits that energy moves from Yin to Yang and Yang to Yin.

The area of the metatarsophalangeal joint of the great toe contains points on the Liver Channel. Manipulation of this area aids in supporting liver function. It should be used with patients suffering with or recuperating from systemic infection, digestive difficulties, or toxicity.

The area of the foot at the metatarsophalangeal joints of the second, third, and fourth digits relates to the Stomach and the Gall Bladder Channels. Manipulation here generally aids the digestive function.

The area of the foot at the metatarsophalangeal joint of the little toe can be used for those who suffer with headache; eyestrain; and upper back, shoulder, and neck tension.

Step 29

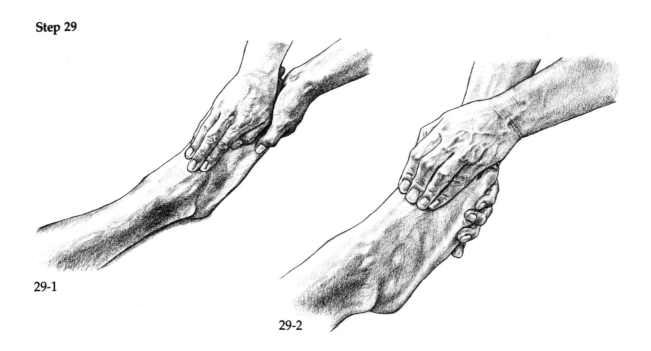

29-1

29-2

30. Using thumb stroking with the left hand, stroke over the most medial aspect of the foot. Begin at the area of the first cuneiform bone and move caudally toward the great toe. As the thumb is placed to begin the stroking movement, note that *the thumb and the thenar eminence mold to the contours of the bony structure of the medial aspect of the foot.*

Areas of the Spleen and Kidney Channels are affected through the treatment of this area. This is useful for patients suffering with gastrointestinal problems, sluggish digestion, flatulence, blood sugar imbalance, and for those who suffer with spinal problems or back pain.

Step 30

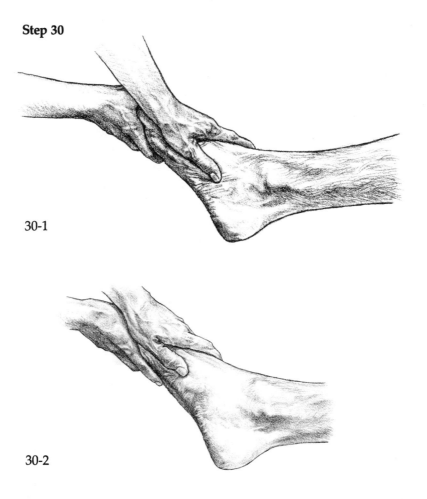

30-1

30-2

This completes the manipulation of the right side of the body. To complete the treatment of the left side of the body, repeat the process, reversing hand directions where necessary. Repetition of the manipulation of the chest and abdomen is recommended.

After completing both sides of the anterior aspect of the body, the Basic Amma continues with the patient lying in the prone position. The practitioner begins the treatment of the posterior surface of the patient's body in a seated position facing the patient's head.

31.   Begin with the hands cupping the upper shoulders with the thumbs lying beside the C7/T 1 area. Using circular thumb pressure, manipulate across the top of the shoulders, in the belly of the upper trapezius, to the lateral edge of the shoulder at the acromio-clavicular joint. A second line of manipulation follows the first, the latter moving along the superior border of the scapula, ending, like the first, at the acromio-clavicular joint. Repeat each line of manipulation five times. One hand works at a time, alternating sides to insure a balanced release of musculature.

Since the hand, not the thumb, is the focus of movement in the administration of this technique, each hand moves in circles that are directed toward the center line of the practitioner's body. In other words, the right hand is moving in a counter-clockwise direction, and the left hand is moving in a clockwise direction. The thumb does not move independently from the movement of the hand itself.

Manipulation here facilitates the release of tension in the upper trapezius. This is very useful with patients suffering with shoulder and neck tension, upper back pain, headache, and impingement of the cervical nerves. Since all Yang channels enter into this region of the body, release of the musculature here will affect Yang energy throughout the body.

Step 31

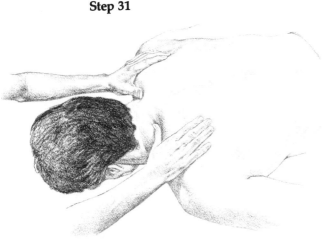

31-1

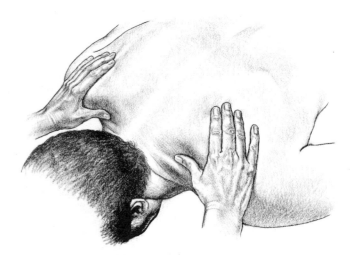

31-2

32. Manipulate around C7/T1, using circular thumb pressure with the arch of the thumb. The right hand works in an arc around one side of the C7/T1 area, and the left hand works in an arc around the other side. Repeat five times. One hand works at a time.

All of the Yang channels of the body cojoin at this area of the body. It tends to be an area of congestion that is notable in the "dowager's hump" frequently exhibited by mature women. The manipulation of this area will aid in the release of this congestion and is also useful in the treatment of headache, back pain, neck and shoulder tension, and pinched nerve.

Step 32

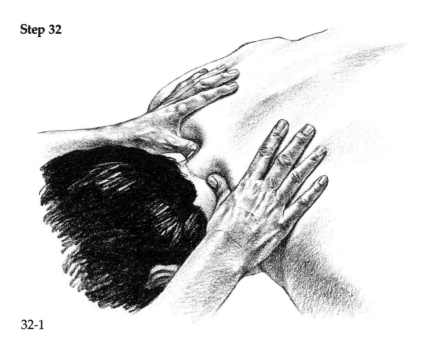

32-1

33. Using circular palmar pressure, work the erector spinae group from the T1 area down to the posterior superior iliac spine (PSIS). This is repeated several times following two specific pathways, each running parallel to the spine. The first pathway lies approximately one inch lateral to the spine. The second lies approximately two inches lateral to the spine, and follows the sagittal plane that lies on the medial border of the scapula, in the lateral border of the erector spinae. The palm

Step 33

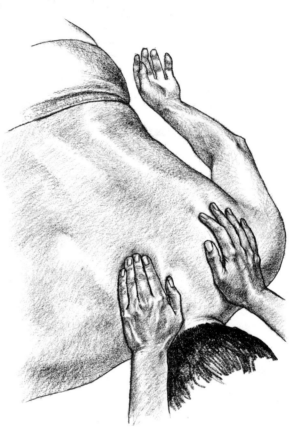

33-1

adheres to the surface of the body during the execution of this technique. Repeat the manipulation of each pathway five times.

The major superficial muscles of the back, the trapezius and the latissimus dorsi, and the deeper erector spinae group, spinalis, longissimus, and iliocostalis are affected in this portion of the treatment.

The area of the manipulation is a portion of the Superficial and Tendino-Muscle aspects of the Bladder Channel. Manipulation of this area is useful for those who suffer with back pain, headache, genitourinary dysfunction, respiratory dysfunction, and cardiovascular dysfunction.

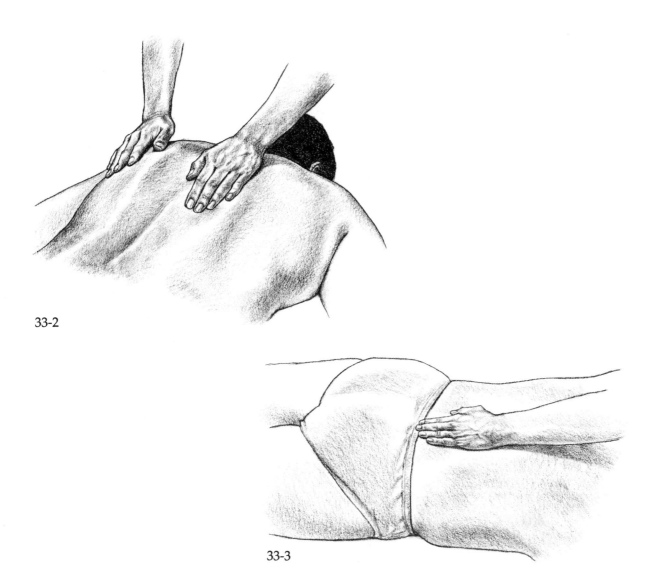

33-2

33-3

34. Using circular palmar pressure, follow the borders of the scapula from the most superior medial edge, around to the most distal, lateral aspect. Use the right hand to manipulate around the patient's right scapula, and the left hand to work around the patient's left scapula. Repeat five times.

This relaxes the trapezius and the latissimus dorsi, as well as the rhomboids and the serratus anterior. This is helpful with patients who experience headache, neck tension, shoulder tension, and upper backache. Patients who suffer with respiratory problems and cardiovascular problems will derive benefit from this manipulation insofar as it serves to release the musculature of the posterior aspect of the thorax, facilitating a free flow of energy in the area.

Step 34

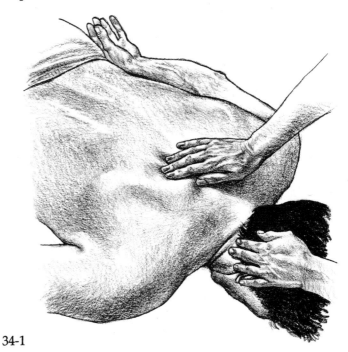

34-1

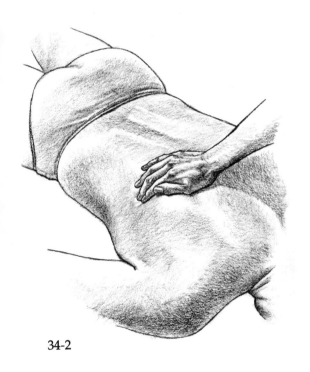

34-2

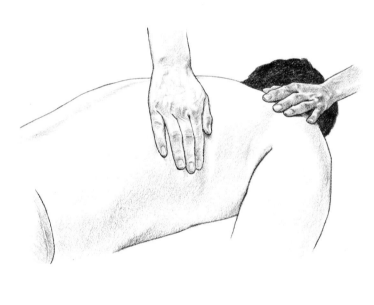

34-3

35. Using palmar stroking with both hands, stroke from the level of C7/ T1 to the PSIS. When the hands reach the PSIS, they rotate with the palm-heel as the pivot point. The return stroke covers the lateral aspects of the thorax. The stroke ends just distal to the axilla. Both hands work simultaneously. Repeat several times.

Step 35

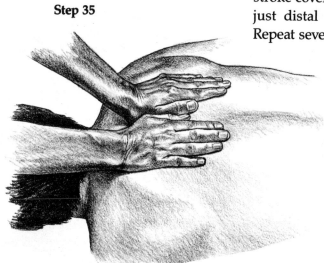

35-1

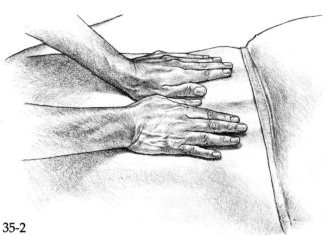

35-2

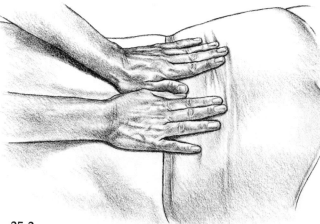

35-3

Stroking in this way relaxes the surface musculature and stimulates the flow of energy in the direction of its patterned flow. This is an extremely beneficial stroke that all patients will find rather soothing.

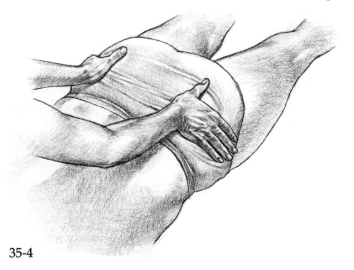

35-4

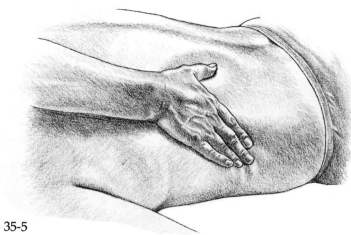

35-5

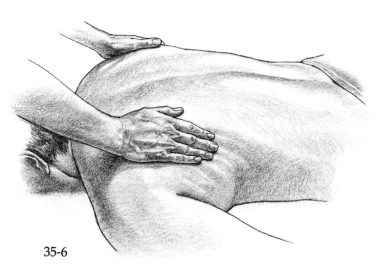

35-6

Move around to the patient's left side.

36. Using circular digital pressure with the right hand, manipulate the sacral area. Begin at the superior border of the sacrum and work down to the level of the coccyx. Be sure to avoid placing any pressure on the coccyx itself. Repeat five times.

In the treatment of this area it is important to remember to respect the patient's privacy. Raise the palm slightly as you move from the superior border of the sacrum to the coccyx in order to avoid direct contact with the gluteal cleft.

This area is an area of concentration of the energy in the Bladder Channel. Problems involving the bladder, kidneys, or genital organs, or any musculo-skeletal problem involving the back, can be helped through the manipulation of this area.

Step 36

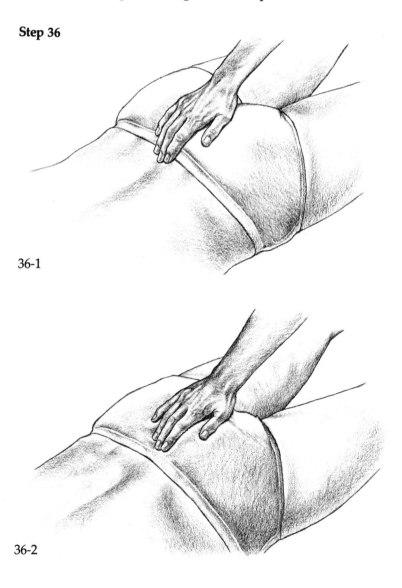

36-1

36-2

37. Using circular digital pressure with the left hand, treat the superior border of the buttock, following the path of the gluteus medius muscle. Begin just superior to the iliac crest and move laterally to the inferior aspect of the buttock at the ilio-tibial tract. Repeat five times.

Step 37

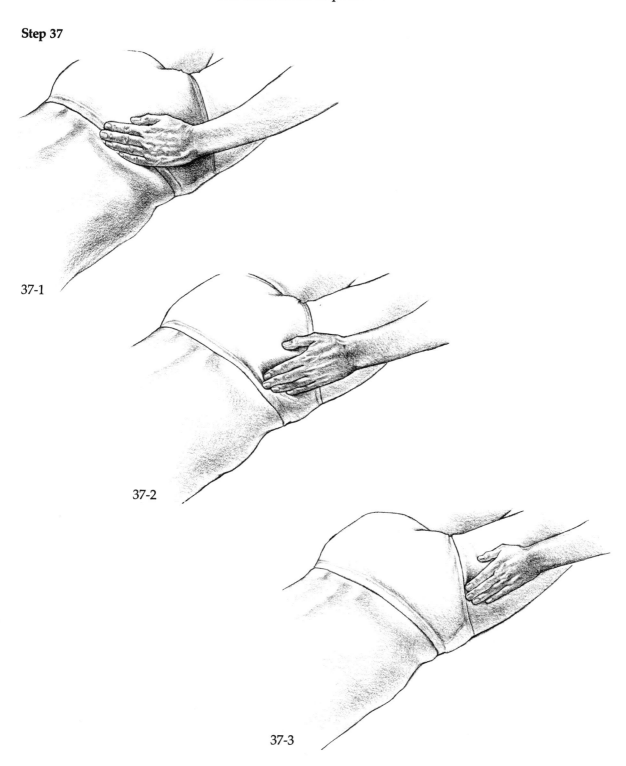

37-1

37-2

37-3

38. Using circular digital pressure with the right hand, manipulate across the gluteus maximus from the PSIS to the center of the posterior thigh at the base of the buttock. Repeat five times.

The manipulation of the gluteal area promotes the relaxation of the entire buttock, the back of the leg, and the lumbar region. It is used with those patients who suffer with back and

Step 38

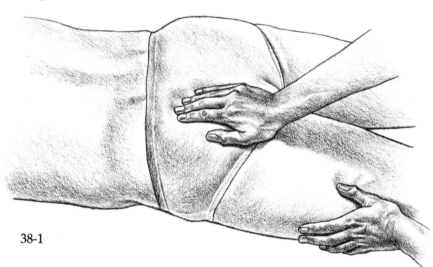

38-1

leg pain. People suffering with degenerative joint disease of the hip and/or knee will experience relief as a result of the manipulation of this area. Joggers and runners often experience pain in these areas. The release of these muscles helps to release leg cramps and prevent their recurrence by increasing the circulation in the legs. Manipulation of this area is also valuable for women who have recently undergone childbirth.

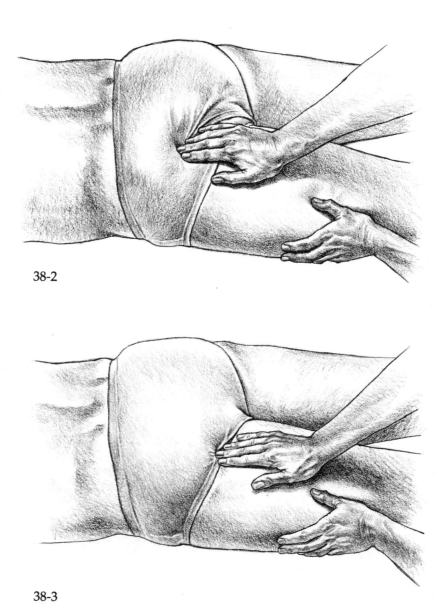

38-2

38-3

39. Using circular palmar pressure with the left hand, treat the lateral aspect of the thigh from the base of the buttock to the knee joint, following the coronal plane. Support the patient's inner thigh with the right hand. Repeat five times.

Step 39

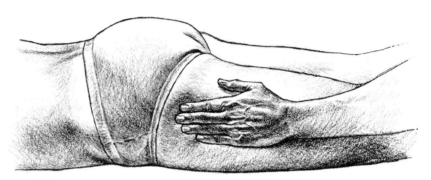

39-1

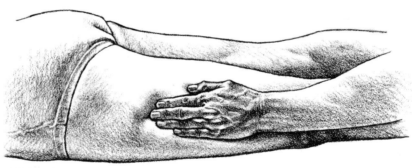

39-2

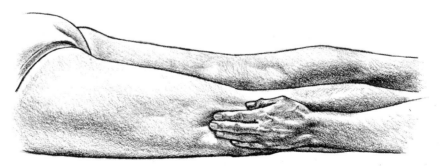

39-3

40. Using circular palmar pressure with the right hand, manipulate the inner (medial) aspect of the thigh from the groin to the knee. Repeat five times.

Treatment of this area relaxes two of the three muscles that constitute the hamstring group—the semitendinosus and semimembranosus, as well as portions of the gracilis and the adductor magnus. Portions of the Kidney Channel lie in this area. Manipulation here is significant in the treatment of genitourinary problems in both males and females, and for people suffering with knee or hip joint pain or injury.

Step 40

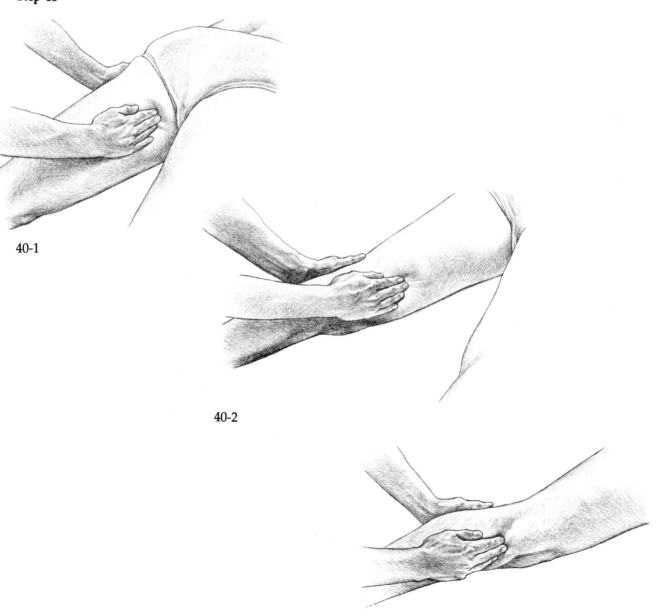

40-1

40-2

40-3

41. Manipulate the center of the posterior thigh, beginning at the base of the buttock and moving distally to the knee. Use circular palmar pressure with the right hand. Support the lateral aspect of the thigh with the left hand. Repeat five times.

Manipulation in this area relaxes the large posterior thigh muscles, the biceps femoris, semitendinosus, and semimembranosus. Manipulation just superior to the popliteal fold will relax the triceps surae of the calf.

In the treatment of this area, portions of the Bladder Channel are affected. This is an area of focus for those patients who suffer with back problems or genitourinary tract dysfunction.

Step 41

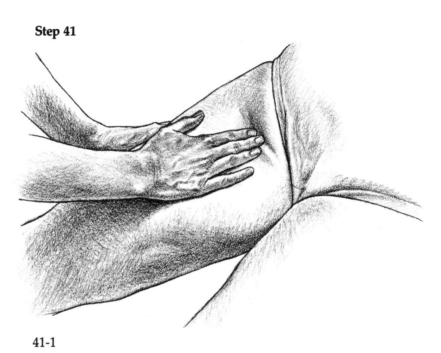

41-1

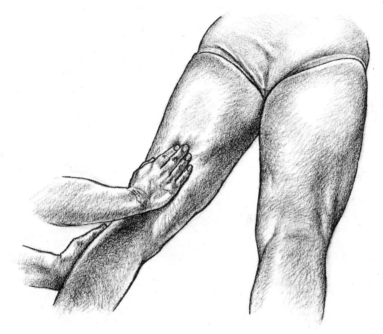

41-2

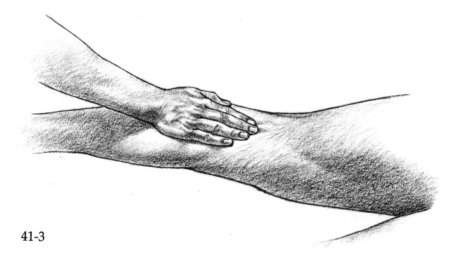

41-3

42. Manipulate the popliteal fold, using circular thumb pressure with the arch of the thumb of the right hand. Support the manipulation by gently grasping the inner knee with the palmar surface of the digits of the working hand. Do not grip the inner knee tightly with the fingers. This tends to be a very sensitive area on many people. A gentle stroke must be used.

The treatment of this area releases the hamstring tendons which insert into this area, thereby relaxing the posterior aspect of the thigh. The musculature of the calf will be affected, as well as the origins of several of the calf muscles.

Two significant Bladder points lie in this area, and it can be an area of focus for patients suffering with back pain, and genitourinary tract dysfunction.

Step 42

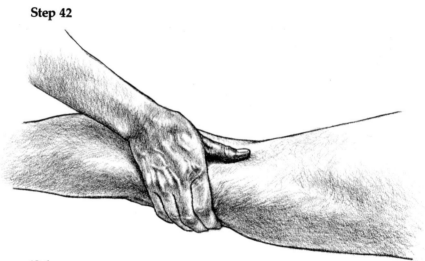

42-1

43. Using thenar embrace, manipulate the musculature of the calf from the back of the knee to the base of the Achilles tendon, ending with thenar embrace to the Achilles tendon.

When thenar embrace is used, the belly of the muscle is drawn into the palm of the working hand. When a practitioner with small hands is working on a patient with large calves, one side of the calf can be manipulated at a time, treating the two bellies of the gastrocnemius muscles independently. Through the manipulation of this area, the entire leg and thigh will relax, as well as the musculature in the lower back and buttocks.

Repeat this entire process to the patient's right side, beginning at the sacral area and working the right buttock and leg.

Step 43

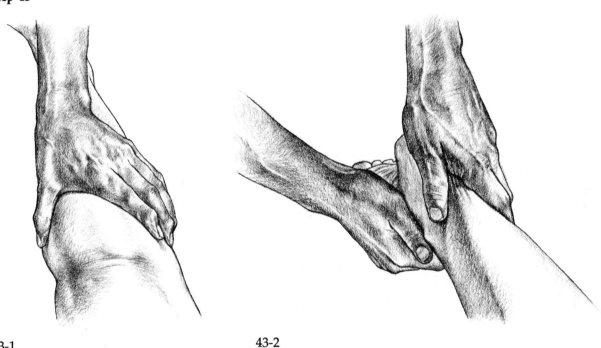

43-1   43-2

Return to a standing position facing the patient's head.

44. Complete the manipulation of the back. Using palmar stroking with both hands, stroke from the level of C7/T1 to the PSIS. When the hands reach the PSIS, rotate the hands using the palm heel as the pivot point. The return stroke will pass over the lateral aspects of the thorax. The stroke ends at the area of the axilla. Both hands work simultaneously. Repeat several times. (See the illustration of Step 35.)

Completion of the treatment in this way serves to completely relax the large muscle groups of the back: the trapezius and the latissimus dorsi. In addition, the manipulation in this direction moves the energy of the Bladder Channel in the direction of its flow.

Step 44   Repeat Step 35

Take a seated position facing the patient's head.

45. Turn the patient's head to *his* right. Treat the area around the ear using circular digital pressure with the distal pads of the digits of the left hand. The middle finger follows the sulcus formed at the squamosal suture. Repeat five times.

Turn the patient's head to his left and repeat the process.

The Superficial and Tendino-Muscle aspects of the Gall Bladder Channel are the focus of treatment. The treatment of this area will relax the patient physically as well as emotionally. There is an emotional component to every disease or ailment. Emotional stress is a part of our daily lives. The release that is resultant from the treatment of this area aids considerably in the attainment of the general state of balance between the body and the mind reflected in what we call well-being.

Step 45

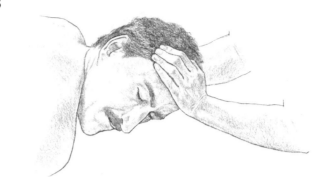

45-1

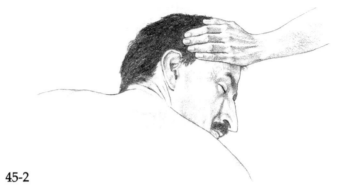

45-2

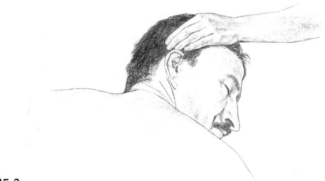

45-3

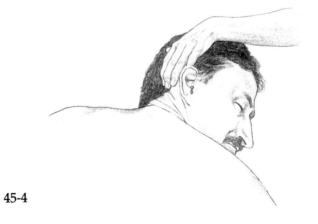

45-4

46. Return the patient's head to the central position. Keeping the fingers of both hands at the base of the occiput, pull up underneath the base of the occiput. Maintain that pressure and then implement circular digital pressure with the distal pads of the four digits of each hand. First direct the pressure into the pads of the fifth digits, and slowly direct the pressure into the fourth, third, and second digits to manipulate the base of the occiput in a lateral-to-medial direction, moving from the ears toward the center of the back of the skull.

Manipulation in this area releases both the superficial and the deeper muscles of the neck: sternocleidomastoid, the upper trapezius, splenius capitis, longissimus capitis, spinalis capitis. Release of these muscles promotes an overall relaxation of the neck, throat, shoulders, and back. Manipulation here is useful for patients suffering with headache, migraine, dizziness, chest tension, and neck, shoulder, and upper back discomfort.

Step 46

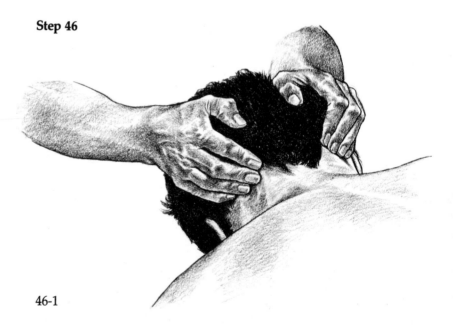

46-1

Repeat the stroking to the patient's back as in Step 44.

Ask the patient to take a seated position. He should be reminded to move slowly to prevent any lightheadedness that may result from sitting up suddenly or quickly.

The practitioner stands behind the seated patient in order to manipulate the posterior aspect of the shoulders and neck.

47. Using thenar embrace, squeeze the upper shoulders, moving the hands from the most medial aspect of the shoulder at the base of the neck to the most lateral aspect. Repeat five times.

Pressure is exerted from the thenar eminence toward the proximal and medial phalanges of the digits of the working hand. To avoid pinching the trapezius, neither the thumbs nor the fingers bend. The manipulation releases tension in the upper trapezius. The release of this muscle is essential for those patients suffering with neck and shoulder tension, cervical nerve impingement, and arthritis or bursitis in the shoulders or the cervical region.

Step 47

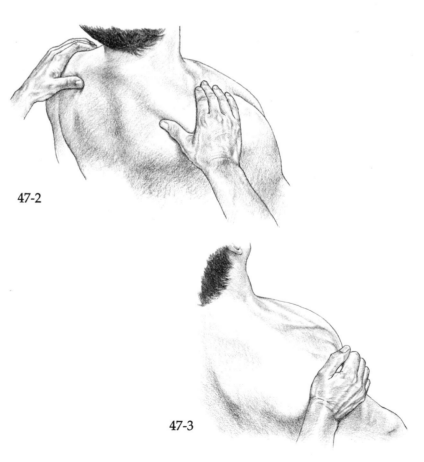

47-1

47-2

47-3

48. Manipulate the uppermost portion of the trapezius muscle, using circular digital pressure. Begin at the base of the neck, with the fingers at the level of C7/T1. Move laterally toward the most lateral aspect of the shoulder at the acromio-clavicular joint. Repeat five times

This is a direct manipulation of the belly of the upper trapezius. Manipulation here effectively releases muscular tension held within this area.

Step 48

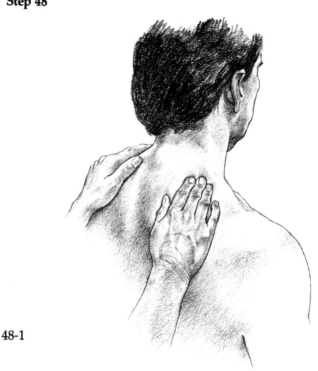

48-1

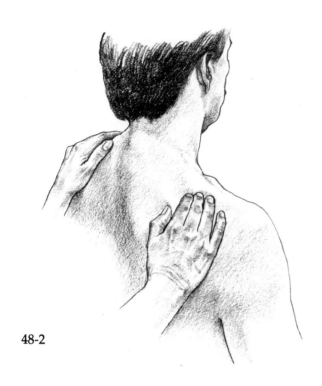

48-2

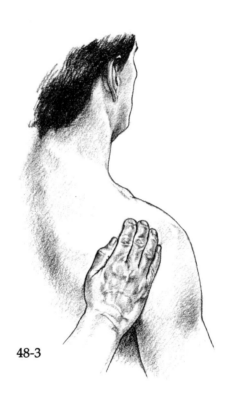

48-3

49. Manipulate the middle portion of the upper trapezius. Begin with the fingers at the level of C7/T1, and using circular digital pressure, work across the superior border of the scapula to the acromio-clavicular joint. Repeat five times.

In addition to the relaxation of the upper trapezius, manipulation across the superior border of the scapula releases the levator scapulae and rhomboid group.

Step 49

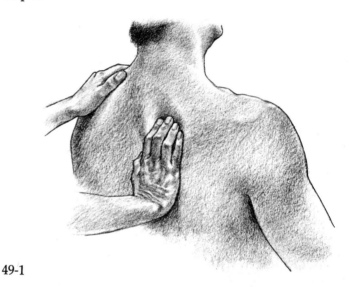

49-1

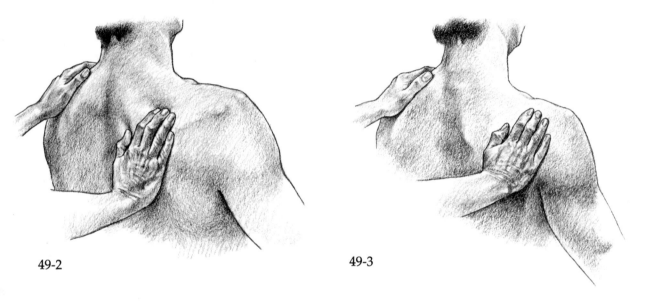

49-2

49-3

Move to the patient's left side.

50. Support the patient's head by allowing him to rest his chin in the palm of the left hand. The tendency will be for the patient to resist complete relaxation of the neck and end up "holding his head." Work with the patient until he is able to let go of the muscle tension and release the complete weight of his head into your hand. As you cup the chin and support the head, you must make sure that the blade of the supporting hand does not rest in the patient's throat.

Manipulate the posterior portion of the right side of the neck with the right hand, using circular digital pressure. Begin the

Step 50

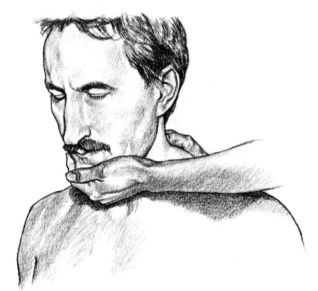

50-1

manipulation at the base of the occiput. Move inferiorly, in the lateral border of the trapezius muscle, toward the top of the shoulder. Repeat five times. Change sides and reverse the process, manipulating with the left hand and supporting the chin with the right.

Supporting the chin allows the patient to completely relax the muscles of the neck. This facilitates the manipulation of the deeper muscles and tendons of the neck, which is essential for patients suffering with cervical arthritis, cervical nerve impingement, and headache resulting from muscular tension. It is through the release of these deeper muscles that vertebral mobility can be improved.

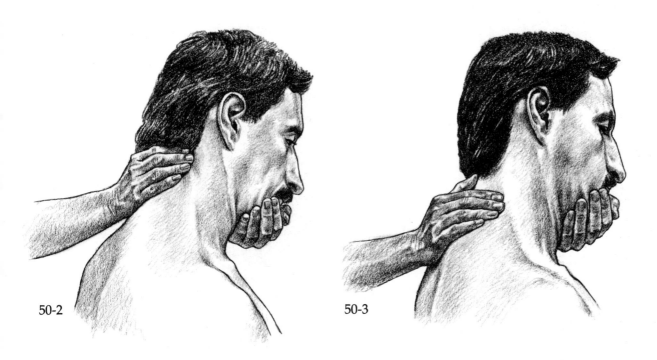

50-2   50-3

51. Continuing to support the chin, use thenar embrace at the back of the neck, gently drawing the musculature posteriorly. Care must be taken to draw, and not squeeze, the musculature of the neck. This generally relaxes the musculature and improves circulation of both blood and lymphatic fluids.

Step 51

51-1

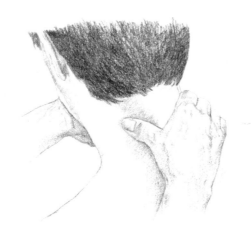

51-2

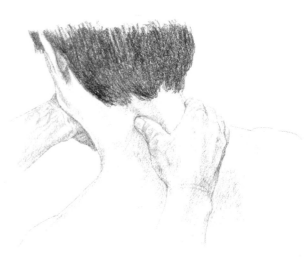

51-3

52. The shoulder manipulation ends with the repetition of thenar embrace to the top of the shoulders, as in Step 47.

Step 52   Repeat Step 47

On the Responsibility of Becoming an Amma Therapist

In wholistic health, "patient responsibility" is a crucial element in the attainment of health. That is, the patient must be completely aware of his role in attaining his health. The professional is a guide; he directs the patient in dietary guidelines, exercise guidelines, and treatment routines. The patient must follow the guidelines provided.

Just so, one who aspires to become an Amma therapist must be willing to take on the responsibility of practicing wholism within his own life—as a *minimal* requirement. The therapist must be in a healthy, balanced physical and emotional condition in order to provide the most beneficial treatments to his patients. Personal health considerations should be used by the therapist toward the development of his own inner harmony and well-being. These include a natural, chemical-free, natural foods diet; an immaculately clean physical body; a program of regular physical exercise, including energy development exercises such as T'ai Chi Chuan and Hatha Yoga; and personal stress reduction measures. Psychological counseling helps the therapist cope with the emotions of day-to-day existence as well as any underlying emotional difficulties that may be experienced.

A therapist is different from a "masseuse." The orientation toward health is different. It is based on concepts of energy movement, balance, and development. For this reason more than any other, the need for balance of the physical, emotional, and intellectual components of the Amma therapist is considered to be absolutely crucial. Once balanced within himself, the Amma therapist can guide another most effectively toward the same kind of balance—that is, health.

Index

INDEX

A

Abdomen, manipulation, 154–57
Accident, and imbalance, 18, 19
Acupressure, 60, 65
Acupuncture, 40–41, 60, 65
Ah shui points, 65–66
Allergies, 142, 148
Anatomical snuffbox, 69
Anatomy
    Chinese medical model, 43–48
    pathways of qi, 62–65
    Western vs. Oriental, 39–42
Ancestral qi, 51
Anxiety, 150
Arm
    absolute yin heart envelope fire
        channel, 57–58, 82–83
    absolute yin tendino-muscle
        channel (pertaining organ—
        heart envelope), 57–58, 102
    bright yang colon metal channel,
        68–69
    bright yang tendino-muscle chan-
        nel (pertaining organ—colon),
        94
    great yang small intestine fire
        channel, 76–77
    great yang tendino-muscle chan-
        nel (pertaining organ—small
        intestine), 98
    great yin lung metal channel, 67
    great yin tendino-muscle channel
        (pertaining organ—lung), 93
    lesser yang san jiao fire channel,
        84–85
    lesser yang tendino-muscle chan-
        nel (pertaining organ—san
        jiao), 103
    lesser yin heart fire channel,
        74–75
    lesser yin tendino-muscle chan-
        nel (pertaining organ—heart),
        97
    manipulation, 149–50
Arthritis, 153, 163, 191
    cervical, 197
Asthma, 148
Austin, Mary, 58

B

Back
    manipulation, 174–77
    pain, 169, 171, 173, 180–81, 186
    problems, 184
    tension, 168
Behaviorism, 8
Bharta Dharma, 60–61
Bioenergy, 60–61
Bladder. *See* Gall bladder; Urinary
    bladder
Bladder-related dysfunctions, 145
Blade, of hand, 121
Blood, 48
    circulation, 198
    creation, 55–56
Blood pressure, 148
Blood sugar, imbalance, 169
Bowels, and viscera, 49–55
Bruxism, 143, 144

Bursitis, 191
Buttocks, manipulation, 178–81

C
Cancer, 24
Cardiovascular problems, 148, 150, 173, 174
Cervical arthritis, 197
Cervical nerve, impingement, 170, 191, 197
Channels
    extraordinary, 91–92
    names, 61–62
    primary organ, 67–89
    tendino-muscle, 93–108
Chest
    manipulation, 154
    tension, 190
Chiao, 44, 47
Chiropractic, 25
Chopping, 133
Circular pressure, hand, 127–30
Circulation, 148, 151, 198
Cleanliness, of therapist, 35
Colds, 142, 148
Colitis, 148, 157
Colon, 156–57
    arm bright yang metal channel, 68–69
    arm bright yang tendino-muscle channel, 94
    and lung, 49–50
Common cold, 142, 148
Conception vessel, 92
Congestion, 142, 144
Constipation, 148, 157
Coughs, 148, 149
Cramps, leg, 181
Creation
    cycle, 45–46
    of energy, pure fluids, and blood, 55–56
Crossing fingers, 125
Cupping, 133, 144
Cutaneous regions, 63, 106–8

D
Deafness, 40, 53
Defensive qi, 48, 50, 65
Depression, 150
Diarrhea, 157
Digestion, 148, 168, 169
Digital pressure, circular, 128
Digital stroking, 131
Direct pressure, hand, 129–30
Disease, 11
    defined, 16n
    iatrogenic, 12
Dizziness, 190
Dowager's hump, 171

E
Education, in wholistic health, 13–14
Eight extraordinary channels, 63
Eight principles, 43
Elements, 44–47
Embracing, 132
Emotional states, 23–25
Emotional stress, 160
Energy, 17–18
    creation, 55–56
    system, 14–15
Environment, and imbalance, 18, 20
Exercise
    hand, 123–26
    and imbalance, 18, 22–23
Exophthalmia, 54
Extraordinary channels, 91–92
Eyestrain, 142, 168

F
Face, thumb stroking, 136–43, 146
Fingers
    crossing, 125
    free edge, 120
    manipulation, 153
    pad, 120
    palmar aspect, 120
    stretch, 123
Fingertips, 124–25
Fist
    loose stroking, 131–32
    stretch, 125
Five elements, 44–47
Five relative phases, 44–47
Flatulence, 156, 157, 169
Flight-fight mechanism, 23
Fluids, pure, creation of, 55–56
Foot
    manipulation, 167–69
    reflexology, 4
Forehead, manipulation, 136–42
Free edge, of finger, 120

G
Gall bladder
    leg lesser yang tendino-muscle channel, 104
    leg lesser yang wood channel, 86–87
    and liver, 54–55
Gastrointestinal disorders, 148, 158
Genital organs, 178
Genitourinary tract
    dysfunction, 167, 173, 183, 184, 186
    infections, 159
Governing vessel, 90–91
GSR (galvanic skin response), 11

H
Hand, 113–20
  anatomical description, 120–21
  care of, 121–22
  circular pressure, 127–30
  crossing fingers, 125
  direct pressure, 129–30
  embracing, 132
  exercises, 123–26
  finger stretch, 123
  fingertips, 124–25
  fist stretch, 125
  manipulation, 151–53
  palmar embrace, 123–24
  percussion, 133
  rolling stones, 125
  stroking, 130–32
  thumbs, rotating, 125
  wrist strengthening, 126
  wrist stretch, 124
Hands-on manipulation, 134–35
Hatha Yoga, 5, 23, 31–32
Head, manipulation, 145, 188–90,
  196–98
Headache, 54, 142, 143, 145, 168,
  170, 171, 173, 174, 190, 197
Healing sensitive, 27–30
Health
  and nutrition, 35
  of therapist, 31–32, 35
Heart
  arm lesser yin fire channel, 74–75
  arm lesser yin tendino-muscle
    channel, 97
  and small intestine, 52
Heart attack, 11
Heart envelope
  arm absolute yin fire channel,
    82–83
  arm absolute yin tendino-muscle
    channel, 102
  and san jiao, 53–54
Heaters, 53–54
Hemorrhoids, 157
Herpes zoster, 41
Hip
  dysfunction, 160, 161–62
  pain, 183
Holism, 15n-16n
Homeodynamic model, 17–25
Homeostasis, 17
Hygiene, 35

I
Imbalance
  external sources, 18–23
  internal sources, 23–25
Iatrogenic disease, 12
Infection, 145, 159
Irritable bowel syndrome, 148

J
Joint diseases, degenerative, 181

K
Kidney, 178
  and bladder, 52–53
  essence, 55
  leg lesser yin tendino-muscle
    channel, 101
  leg lesser yin water channel,
    80–81
Knee
  dysfunction, 160, 161–62
  manipulation, 186–87
  pain, 183
Ku qi, 48

L
Leg, 163–66
  absolute yin liver wood channel,
    88–89
  absolute yin tendino-muscle
    channel (pertaining organ—
    liver), 105
  bright yang stomach earth chan-
    nel, 70–71
  bright yang tendino-muscle chan-
    nel (pertaining organ—
    stomach), 95
  great yang tendino-muscle chan-
    nel (pertaining organ—urinary
    bladder), 99–100
  great yang urinary bladder water
    channel, 78–79
  great yin spleen earth channel,
    72–73
  great yin tendino-muscle channel
    (pertaining organ—spleen), 96
  lesser yang gall bladder wood
    channel, 86–87
  lesser yang tendino-muscle chan-
    nel (pertaining organ—gall
    bladder), 104
  lesser yin kidney water channel,
    80–81
  lesser yin tendino-muscle chan-
    nel (pertaining organ—
    kidney), 101
  pain, 180–81
  and thigh, 158–66
Life, 11
Life energy, 4–5, 6n
Liver
  and gall bladder, 54–55
  leg absolute yin tendino-muscle
    channel, 105
  leg absolute yin wood channel,
    88–89

Lung, 149
    arm great yin metal channel, 67
    arm great yin tendino-muscle
        channel, 93
    and colon, 49–50
Lymphatic fluids, circulation, 198
Lymph nodes, 159

M
Manipulation, 32, 134–35
Massage, 26–27
    therapeutic, 4
Medication, and imbalance, 21–22
Menstrual problems, 145
Microorganisms, and imbalance,
        18, 22
Middle qi, 50
Migraine, 190
Mindbody, 11–12
Mononucleosis, 24
Mucus, 146
Muscular strength, 117–18
Musculo-skeletal difficulties, 23,
        24–25

N
Neck
    discomfort, 190
    manipulation, 144, 191, 196–98
    tension, 168, 170, 171, 174, 191
Nerve, pinched, 171
New Center for Wholistic Health
        Education and Research, 6
Nutrient cycle, 62
Nutrient qi, 50, 56, 65
Nutrition, and imbalance, 18,
        20–22

O
Orbs, functional, 49–55

P
Pad, of finger, 120
Palm, of hand, 121
Palmar aspect, finger, 120
Palmar embrace, 123–24, 132
Palmar pressure, circular, 128
Palmar stroking, full, 131
Palm-heel of hand, 121
    circular pressure, 129
Palpation, 118–19, 140, 145
Pathways of qi
    anatomy, 62–65
    names, 56–59
    for therapist, 60–66
Percussion, 133
Pernicious influences, 20
Physician, health of, 13
Physics, 7–8
    subatomic, 15

Physiological malfunction, and
        imbalance, 23, 24
Physiology, Oriental, 49–55
Pinched nerve, 171
Pneumonia, 148
Porket, Manfred, 42
Prenatal qi, 47–48, 55
Pressure
    circular, 127–29
    direct, 129–30
Pressure points, 65–66
Preventive medicine, 14
Primary organ channels, 63, 67–89
Prostatic disorders, 145
Psychology, 8–9
Pure fluids, creation, 55–56

Q
Qi, blood, and fluids, 47–48
    see also Pathways of qi

R
Reductionism, 9–10
Reich, Wilhelm, 61
Relaxation, hand and body, 116–17
Relative phases, 44–47
Respiratory problems, 173, 174
Rhinitis, 146
Richenbacker, Baron Von, 61

S
San jiao, 58–59
    arm lesser yang fire channel,
        84–85
    arm lesser yang tendino-muscle
        channel, 103
Self-awareness, 33–34
Sensitivity, 5
Sheldon, W., 24
Shoulder, 170–73
    discomfort, 190
    manipulation, 191–95
    tension, 168, 170, 171, 174, 191
Sinus headache, 142, 146
Six chiao, 44, 47
Six pernicious influences, 20
Skeletal alignment, 117
Small intestine
    arm great yang fire channel,
        76–77
    arm great yang tendino-muscle
        channel, 98
    and heart, 52
Smoking, 149
Sohn, Robert, 30
Sohn, Tina, 6, 28–30, 64, 114, 116
Spinal problems, 169
Spleen, 41–42
    leg great yin earth channel,
        72–73

Spleen (*continued*)
  leg great yin tendino-muscle
    channel, 96
  and stomach, 50–51
Sternal area, manipulation, 147–48
Stomach
  leg bright yang earth channel,
    70–71
  leg bright yang tendino-muscle
    channel, 95
  and spleen, 50–51
Strength, of therapist, 31
Stroking, 130–32
Systemic infection, 159, 168

T
T'ai Chi Chuan, 5, 23, 24–25, 33
Tao, 11
Temple, manipulation, 143
Temporomandibular joint syn-
    drome, 143
Tendino-muscle channels, 63,
    64–65, 93–108
Tension, 143, 144, 145
Thenar embrace, 132
Therapeutic massage, 4
Therapist, 26–27
  healing sensitive, 27–30
  health, and nutrition, 35
  as model, 13
  pathways of qi for, 60–65
  self-awareness, 33–34
  training, 5, 30–35
Therapy, 3–6
Thigh, 158–62
  manipulation, 182–85
Three heaters, 53–54
Thumb, 121
  circular pressure, 127–28
  rotating, 125
Thumb stroking, 131
  face, 136–43, 146
Torso, and hands, 115

Toxicity, 168
Training, therapist, 5, 30–35
Treatment principles, 134–35
Trigger point therapy, 65
Twelve cutaneous regions, 63
Types, study of, 24

U
Ulcer, 157
Ulnar aspect, of hand, 121
Ulnar circular pressure, 129
Upper back
  discomfort, 190
  pain, 170, 174
  tension, 168
Upper body, and hands, 115
Upper chest, manipulation, 148
Urinary bladder, 178
  and kidney, 52–53
  leg great yang tendino-muscle
    channel, 99–100
  leg great yang water channel,
    78–79

V
Viscera, and bowels, 49–55
Voll, R. Reinhold, 51, 58, 59, 64

W
Wei qi, 50
Wholism, 10
Wholistic Health Center, 5, 6
Wrist
  strengthening, 126
  stretch, 124

Y
Yin and Yang, 43–44, 63–64
Yuan qi, 55–56

Notes

Notes

Notes

Notes